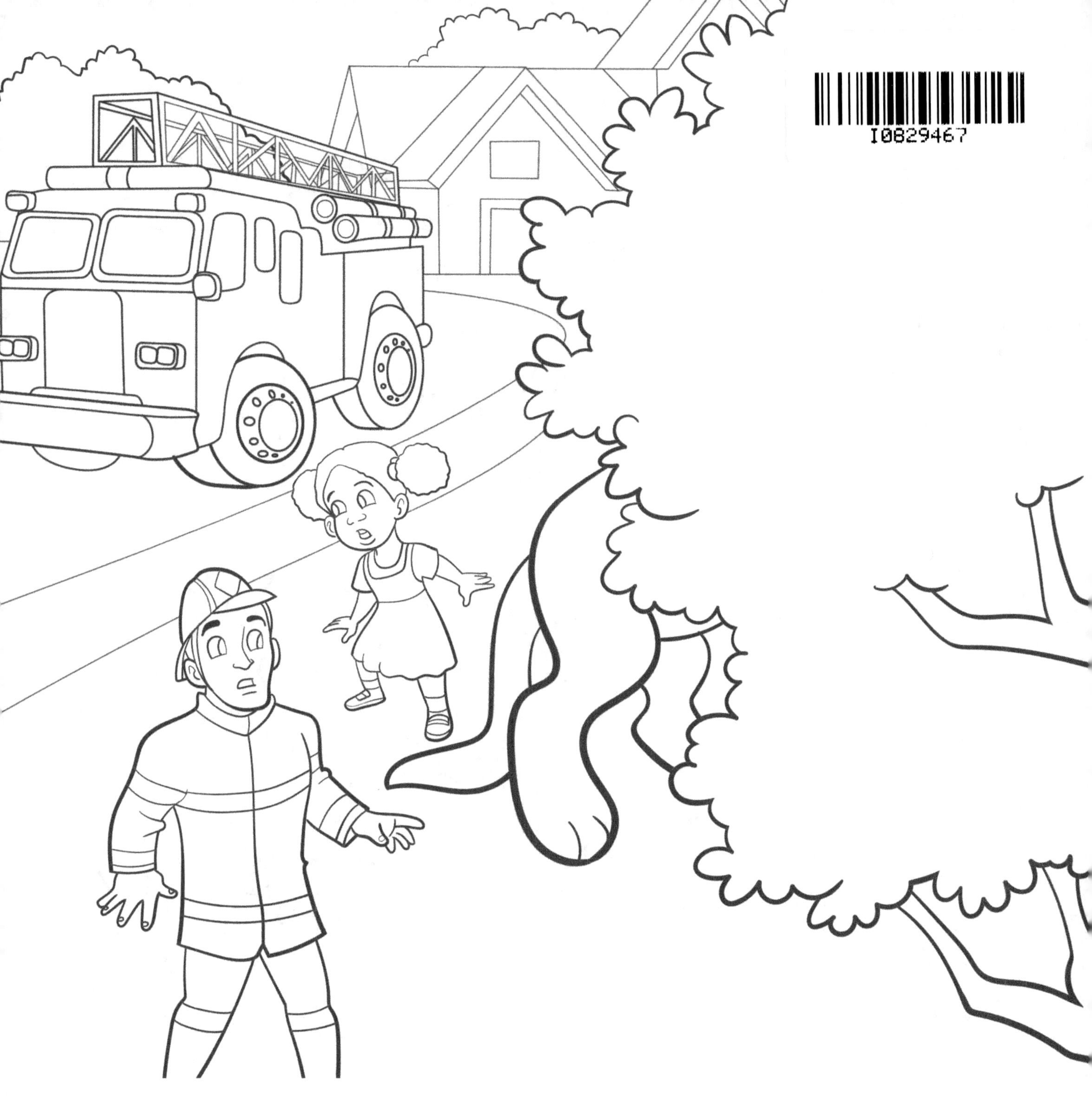

As the fire truck arrives at 420 Place, the fireman looks up. And sure enough, there is a big green cat stuck way up high in the top of the tree.

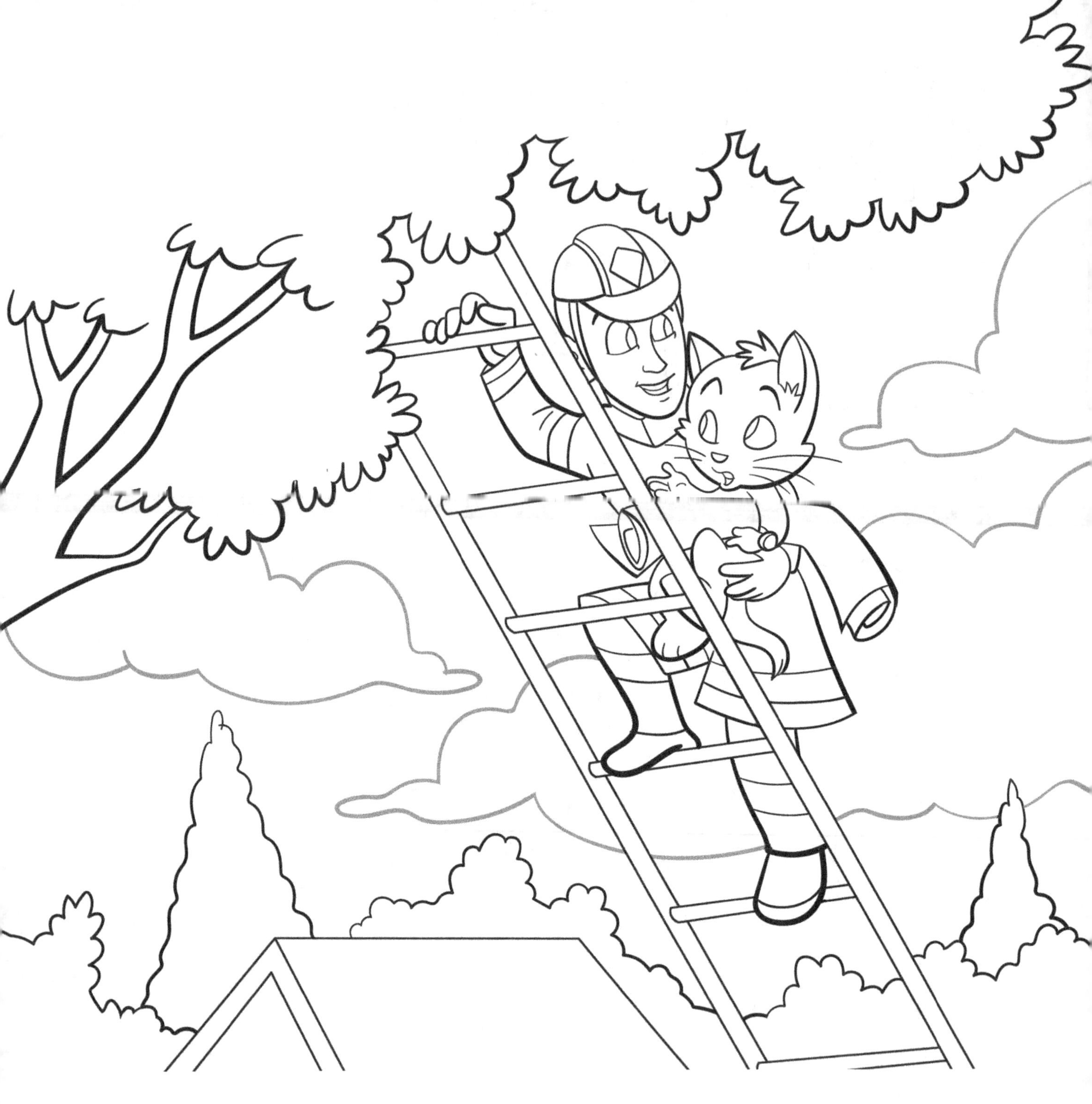

"Thank you for saving me!" says the cat with an innocent smile. "My name is Cannabis. I am Cannabis the Cat!

Cannabis The Cat
To The Rescue
COLORING BOOK

Written by
Jerry Frye

Illustrations by
Mike Motz

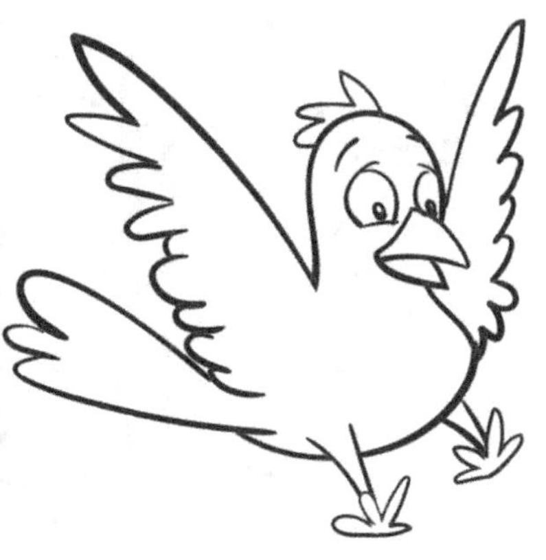

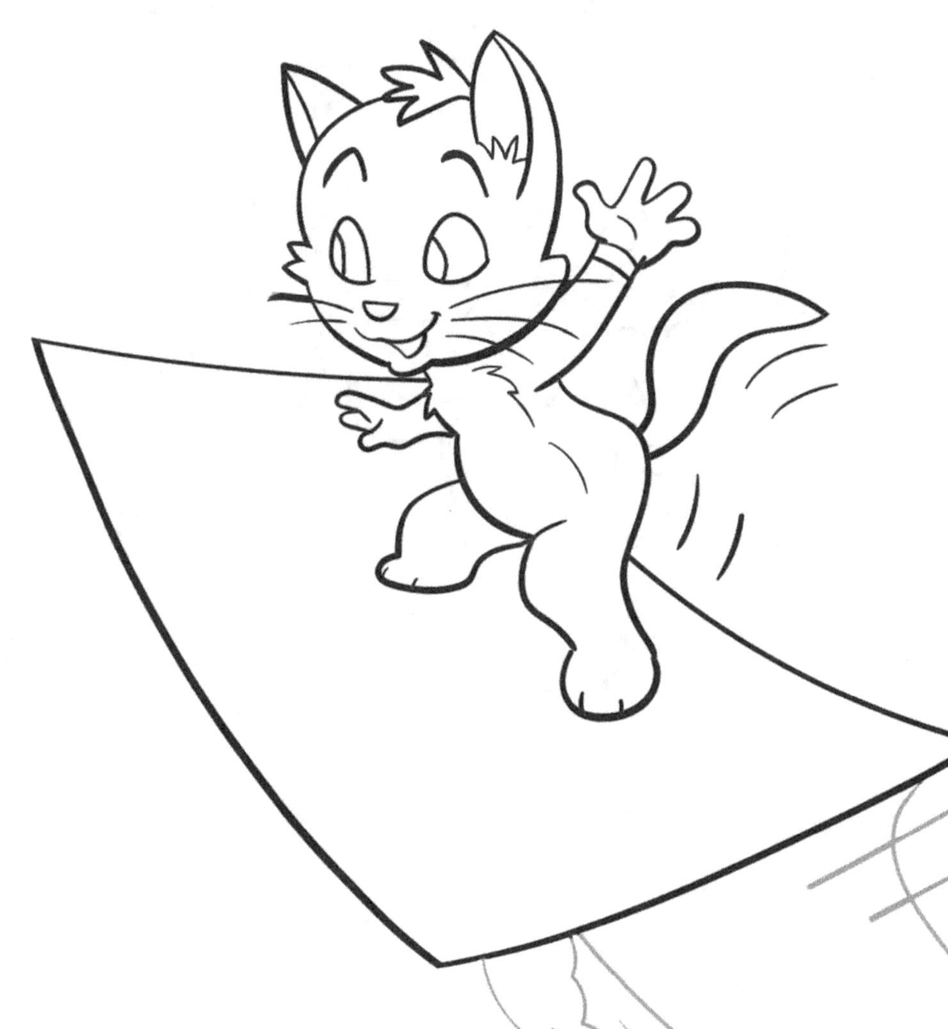

Visit Cannabis online at:
Cannabisthecat.com

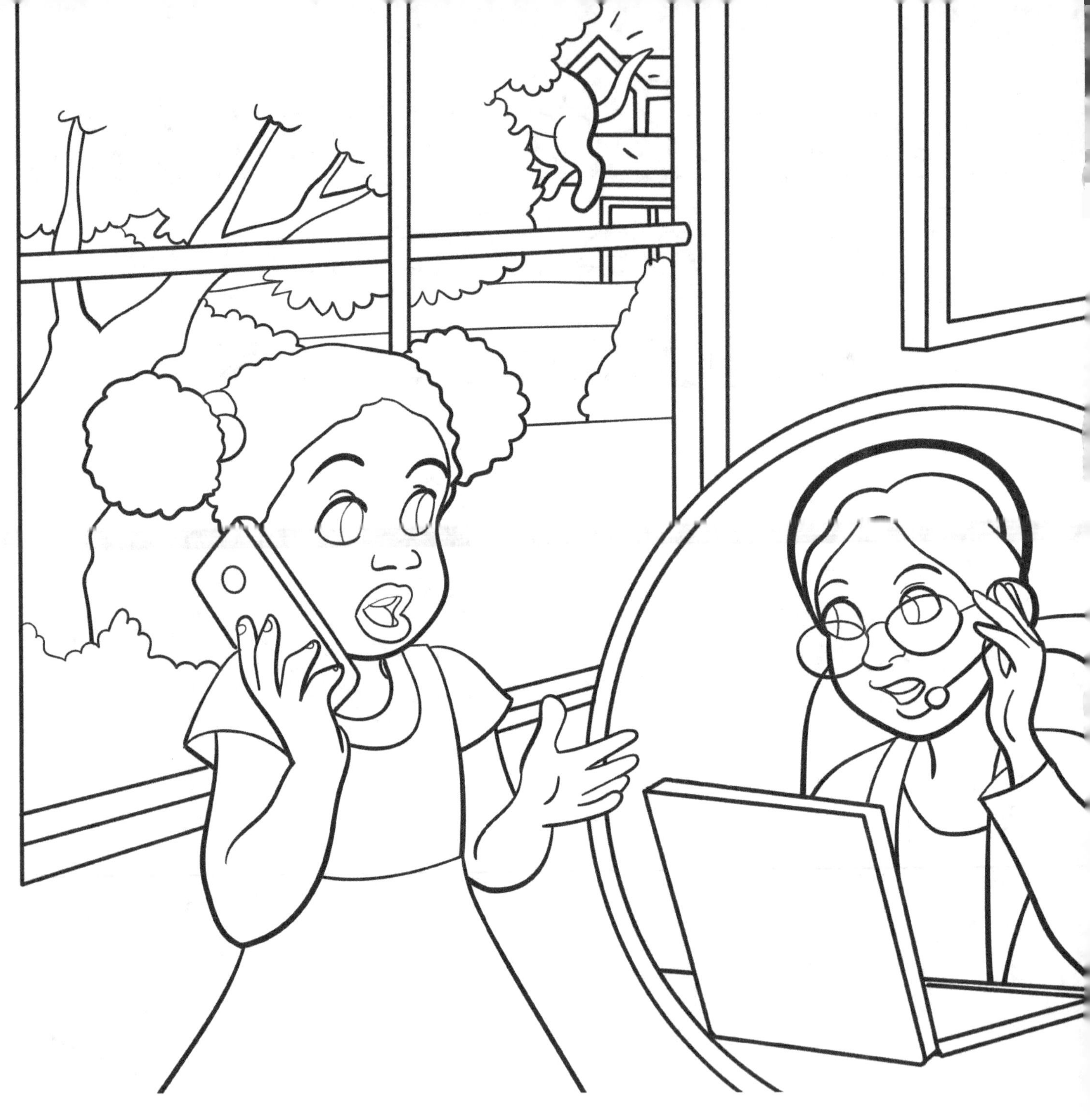

"My name is Nevaeha, my big green cat is stuck way high up in the tree. My address is 420 Place. Please hurry fast!"

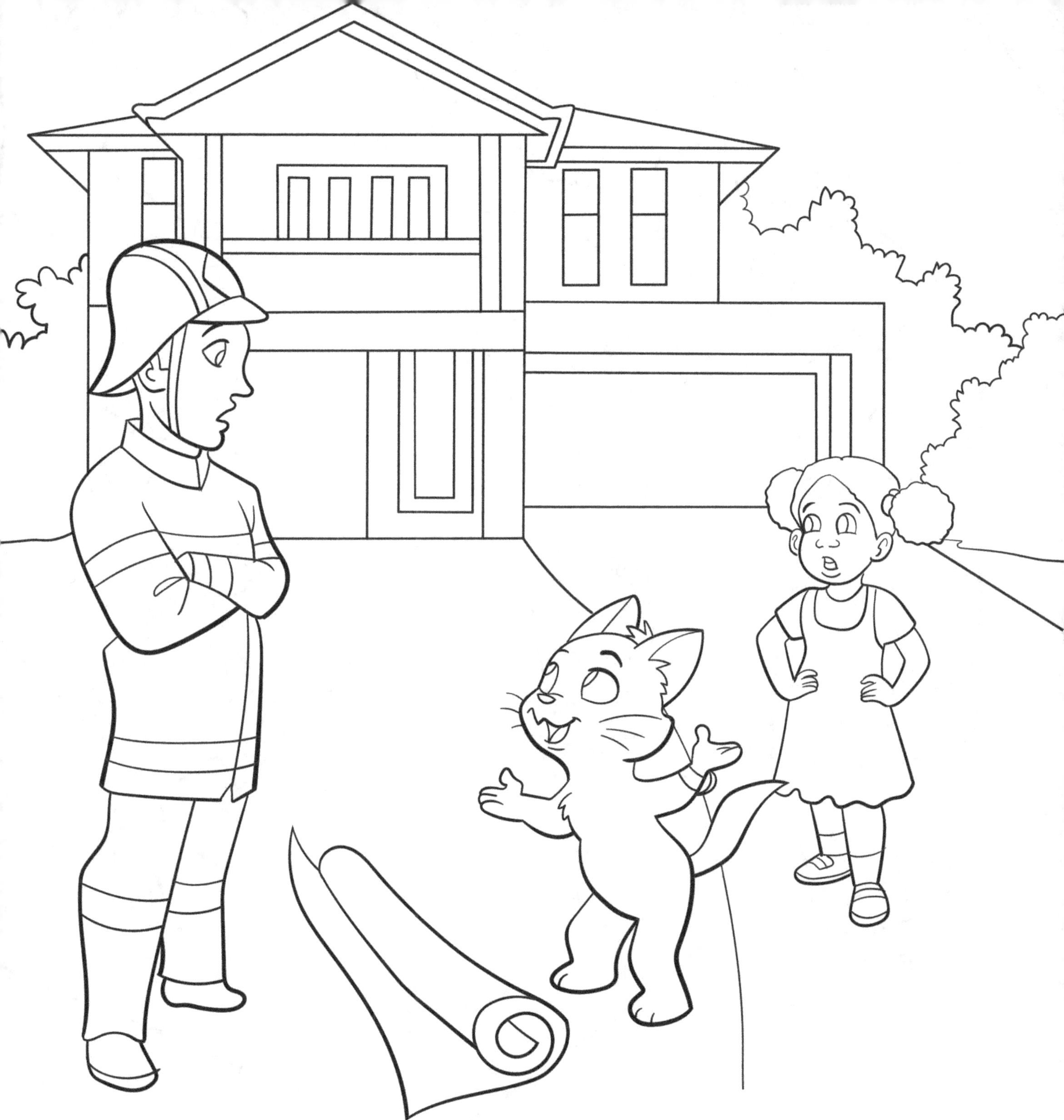

"I was flying perfectly fine on my magic hemp carpet. Then suddenly it became very windy. Before I knew it, I crashed into this big tall tree," says Cannabis.

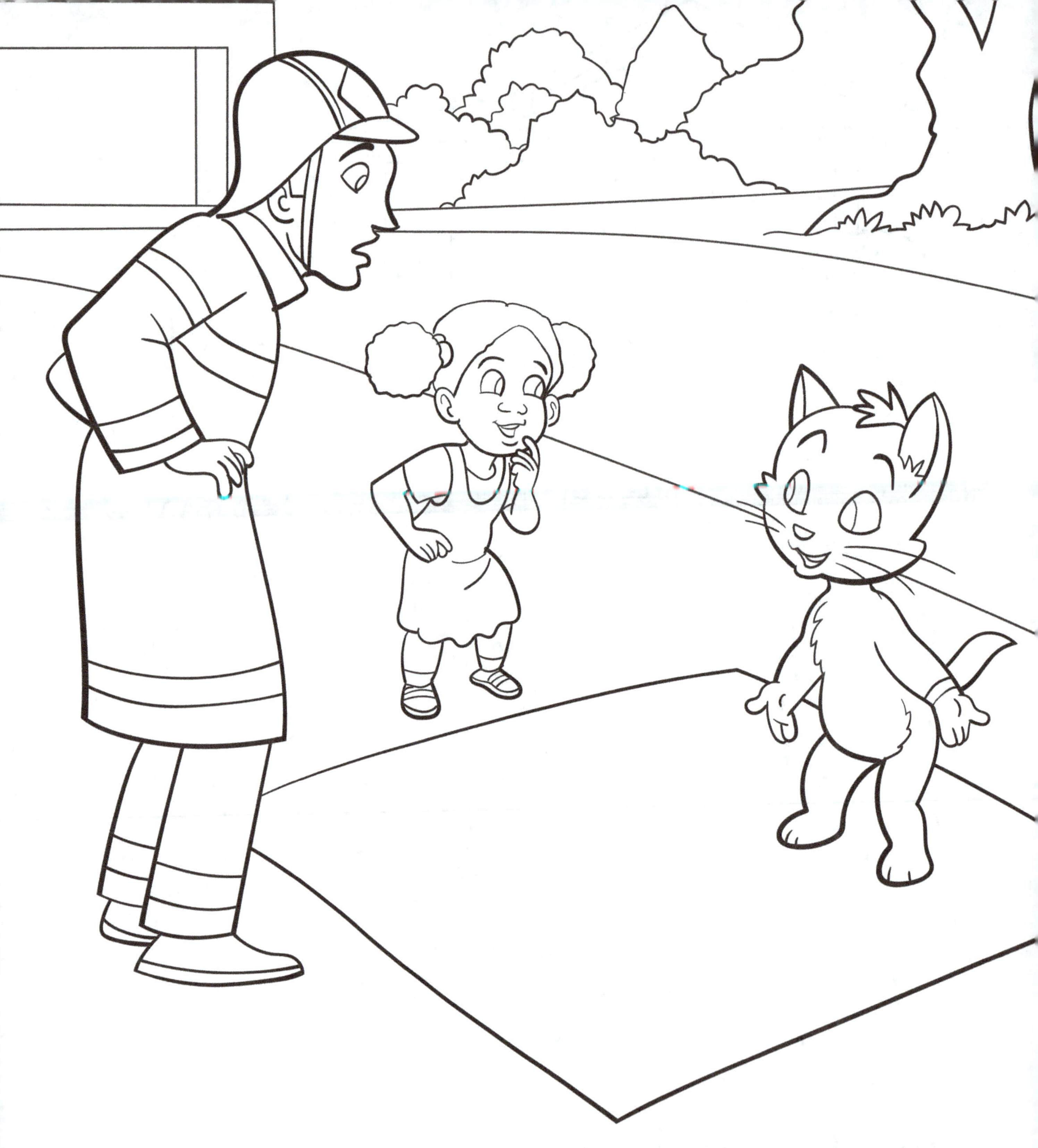

"Your magic hemp carpet?" gasps Jerry.
"Yes! I have a magic hemp carpet that allows me to fly across the sky," says Cannabis.

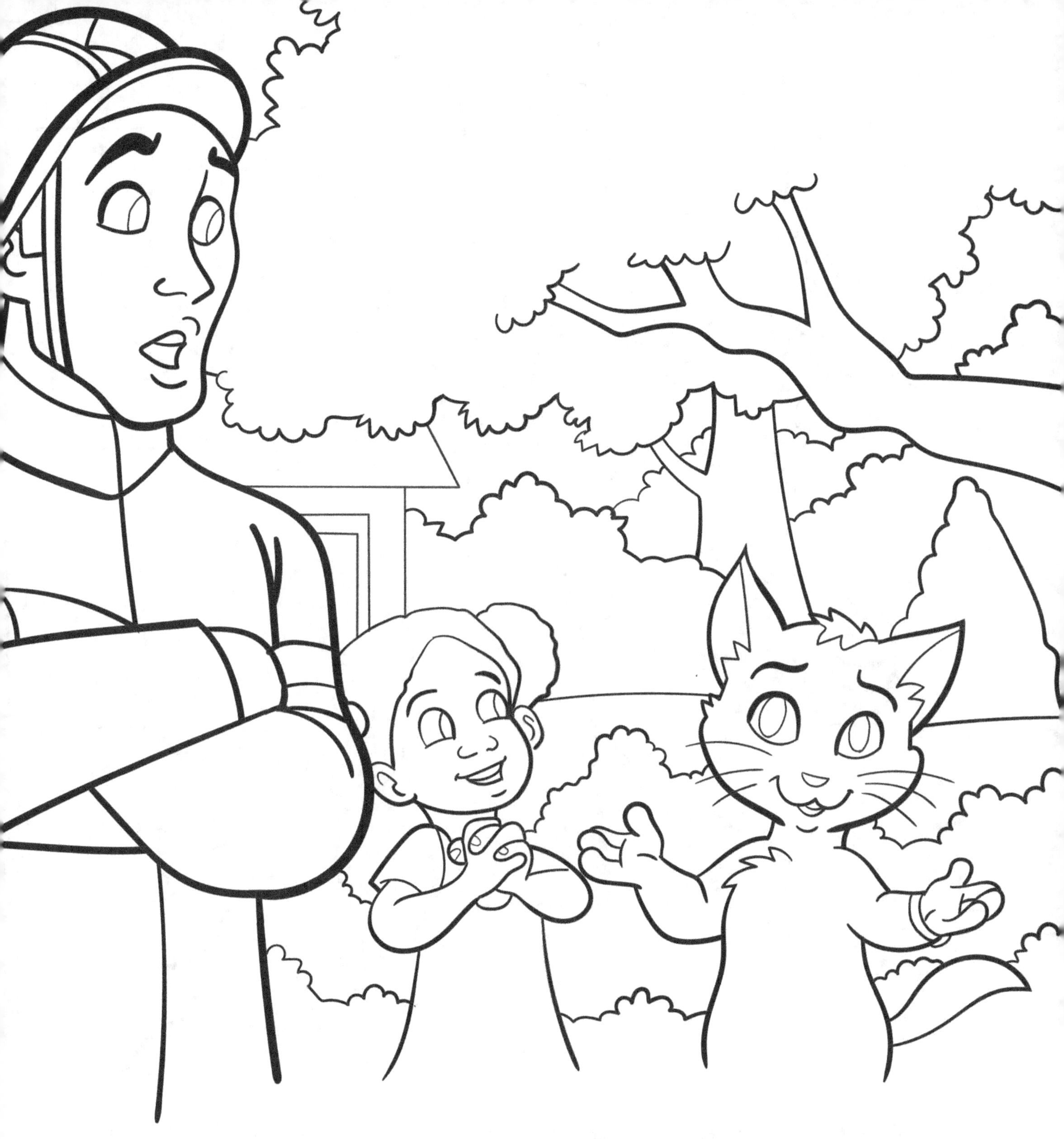

"If someone has a Cannabis emergency, they dial 420 and I respond," says Cannabis.

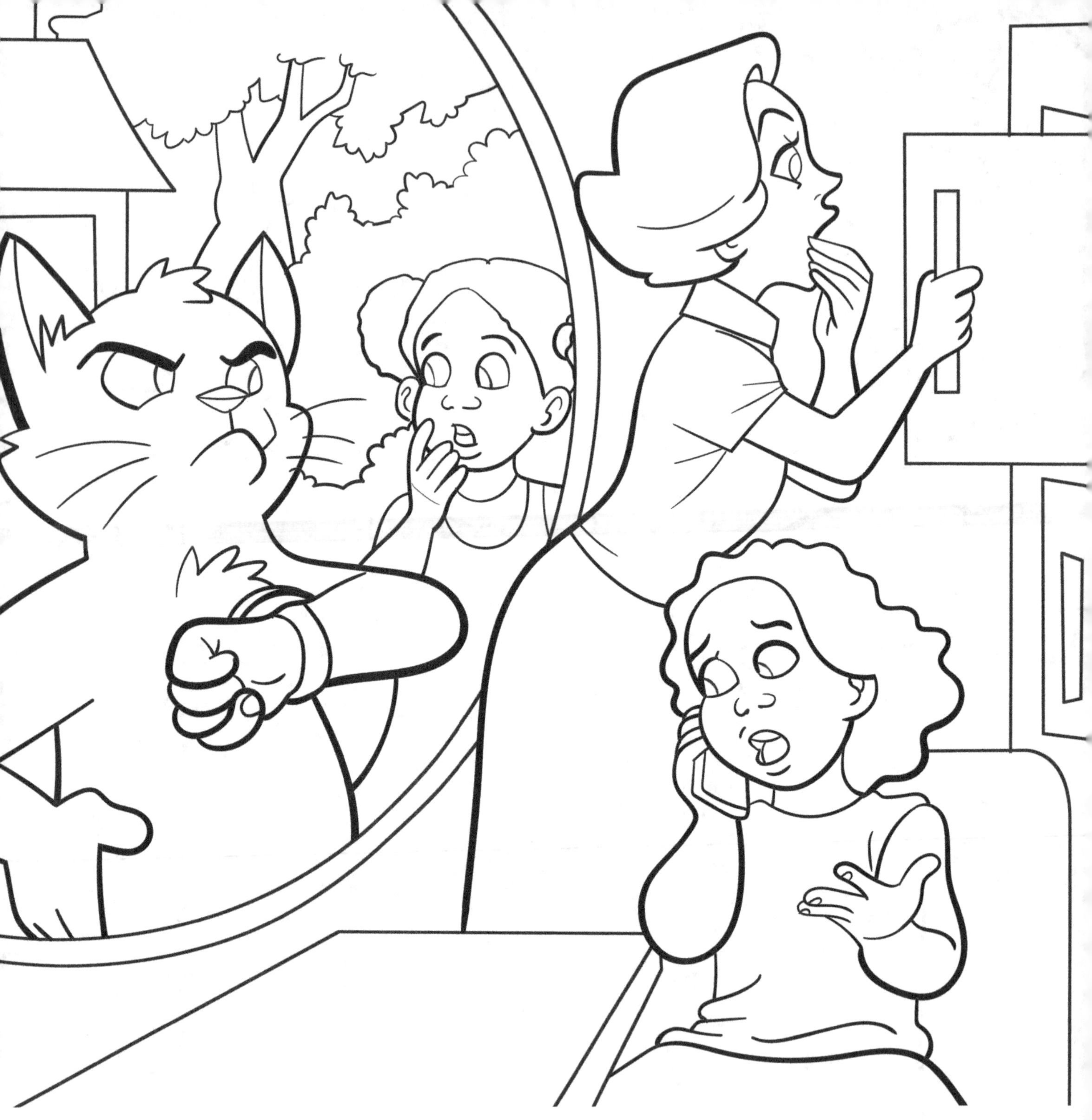

Suddenly, Cannabis's watch lights up. "Hello, this is Cannabis the Cat. What's your 420 emergency?"

"My name is Charlotte. I'm in third grade, and the nurse cannot find my CBD oil.   I'm afraid I'll have a seizure. Can you help me get some CBD oil?"

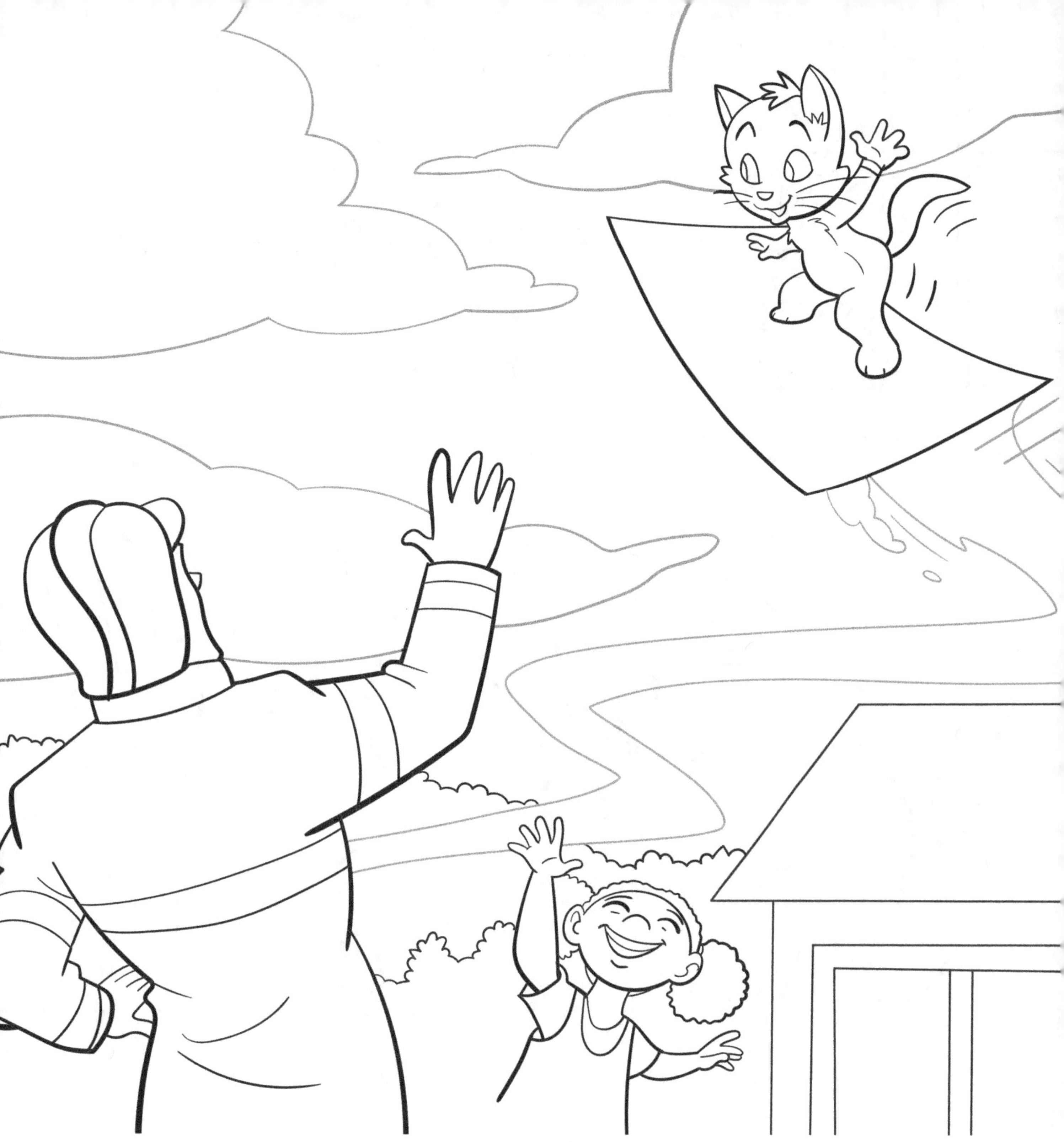

"Yes, of course," says Cannabis. "I'll be right there."
Cannabis says goodbye to his friends and flies off for
Charlotte's school.

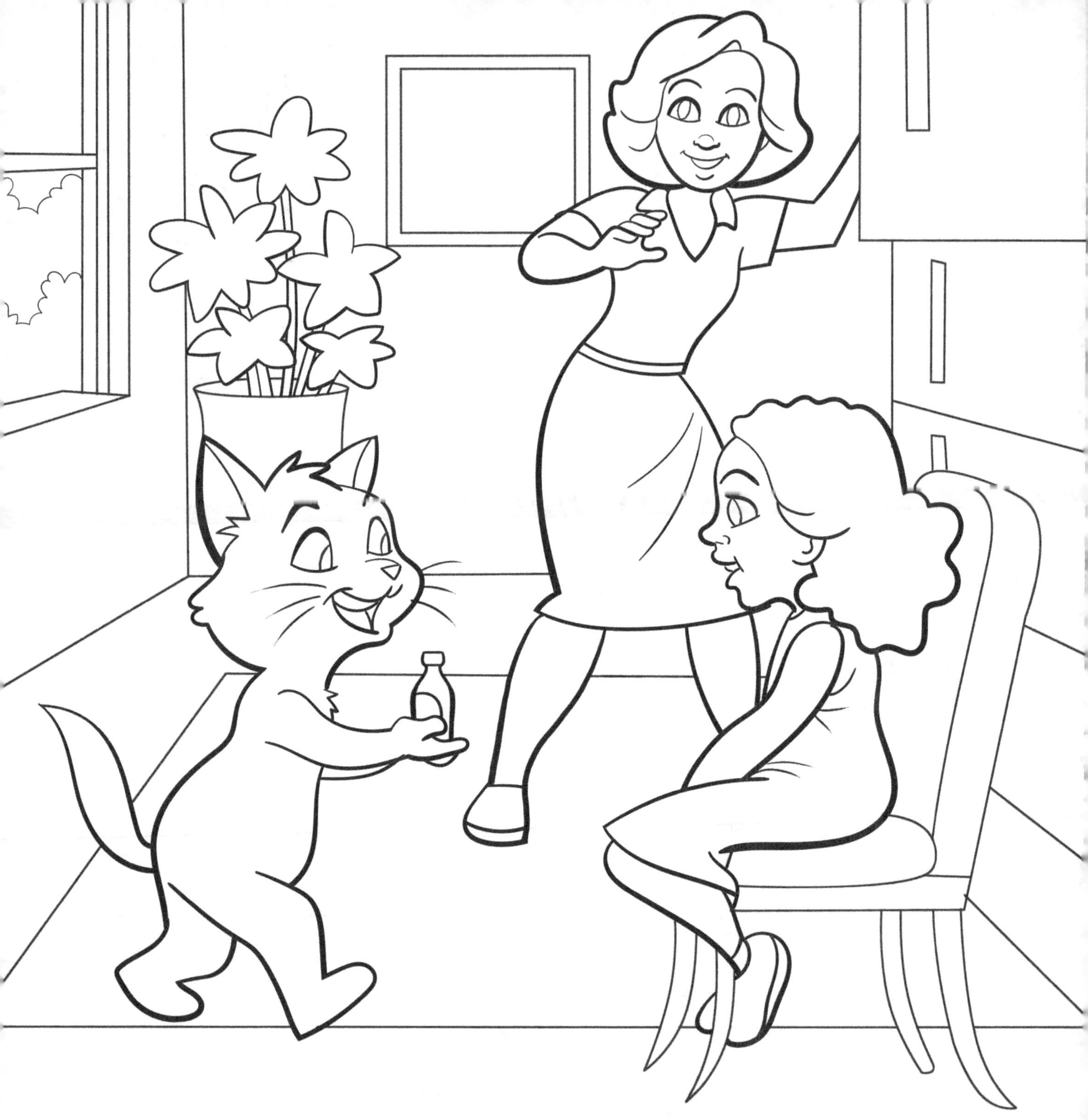

"I brought you FDA-approved CBD oil. This CBD oil will help you remain seizure free. CBD stands for cannabidiol and is one of the main active ingredients in the hemp plant," says Cannabis.

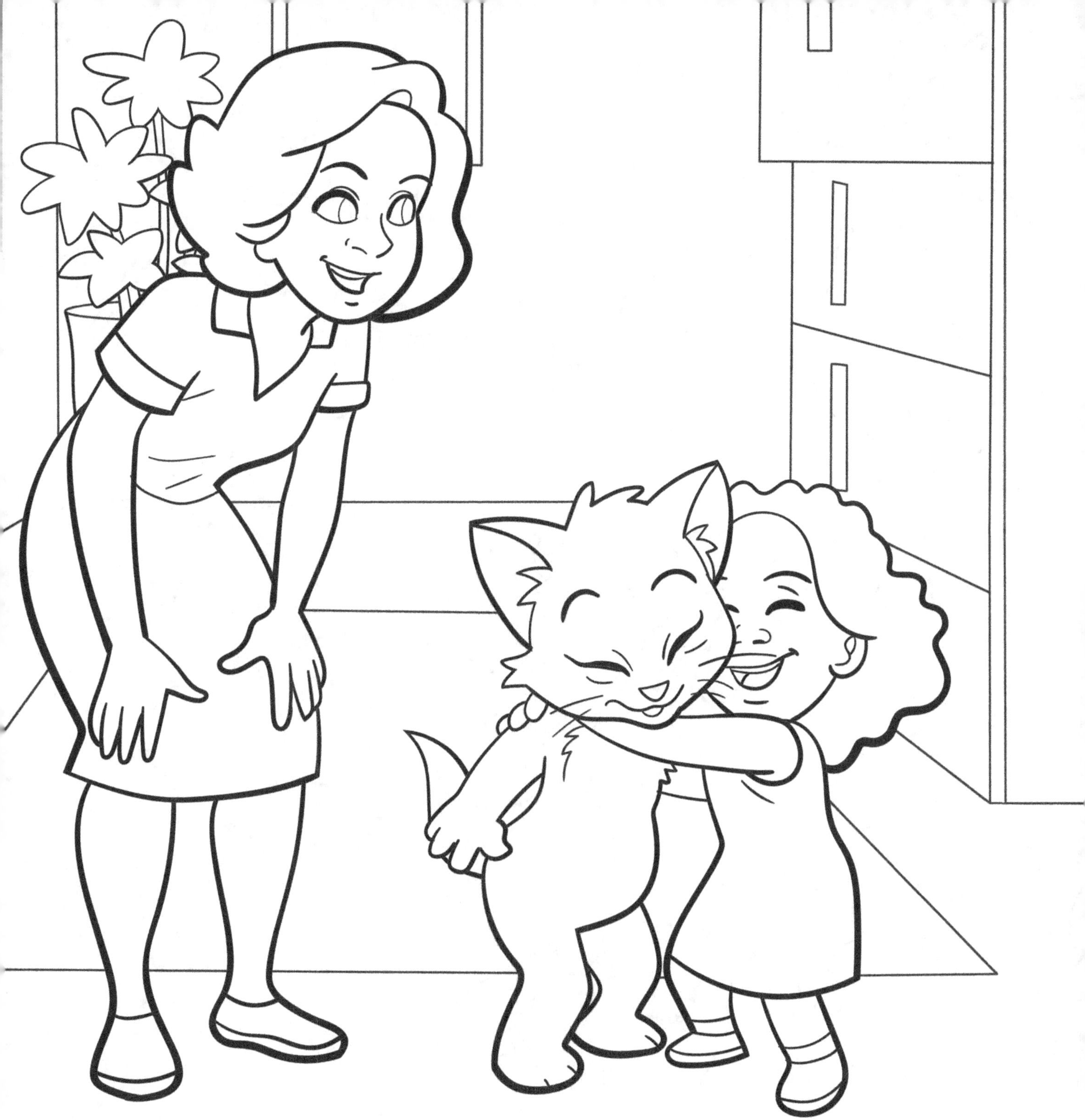

"Thanks, Cannabis. Ever since I began taking CBD oil, I have been seizure free. You're my hero." Charlotte gives Cannabis a big hug and says goodbye.

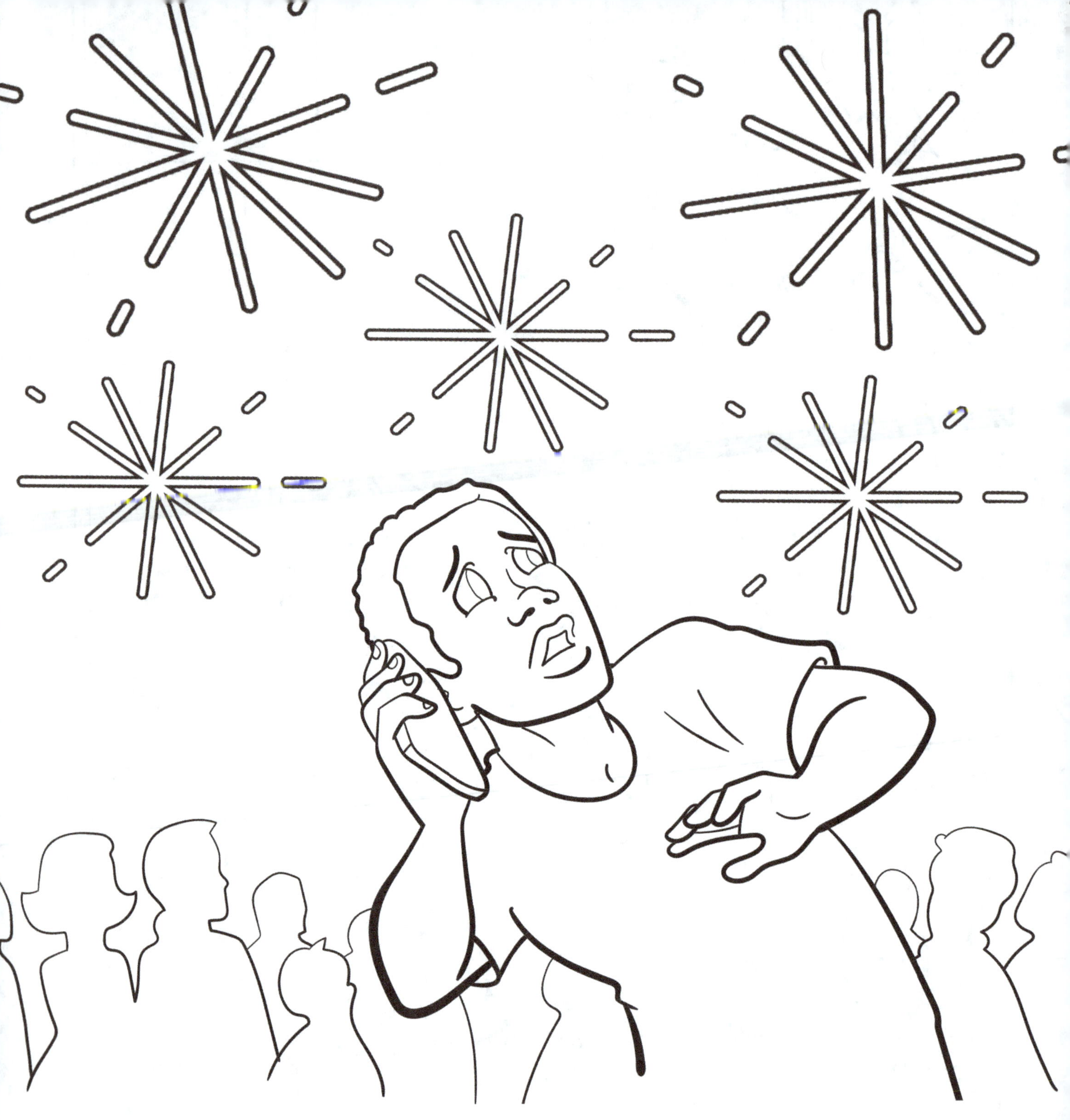

Minutes later, Cannabis's 420 watch goes off. Instantly, he jumps to his feet and springs into action! "Cannabis the Cat, what's your 420 emergency?"

"Hello, my name is Devon. I am a veteran of the U.S. Army, and I suffer from PTSD.

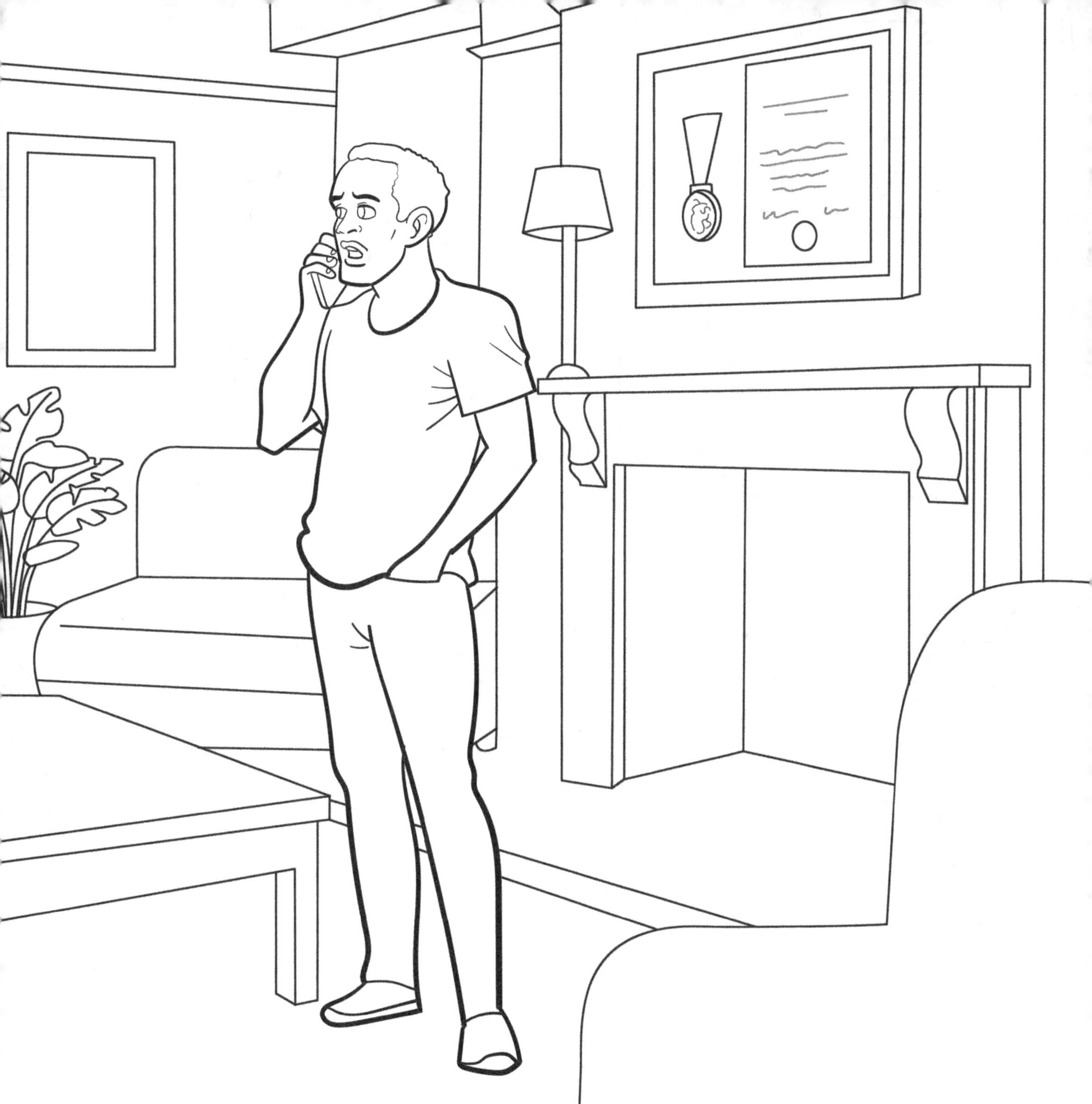

"The VA doctor is not allowed to even talk to me about marijuana. All they want to do is prescribe me pills. I'm afraid I'll become addicted to those pain pills. Can you help me find some high-level THC marijuana?" asks Devon.

"Yes of course," replies Cannabis. "I'm on my way!"

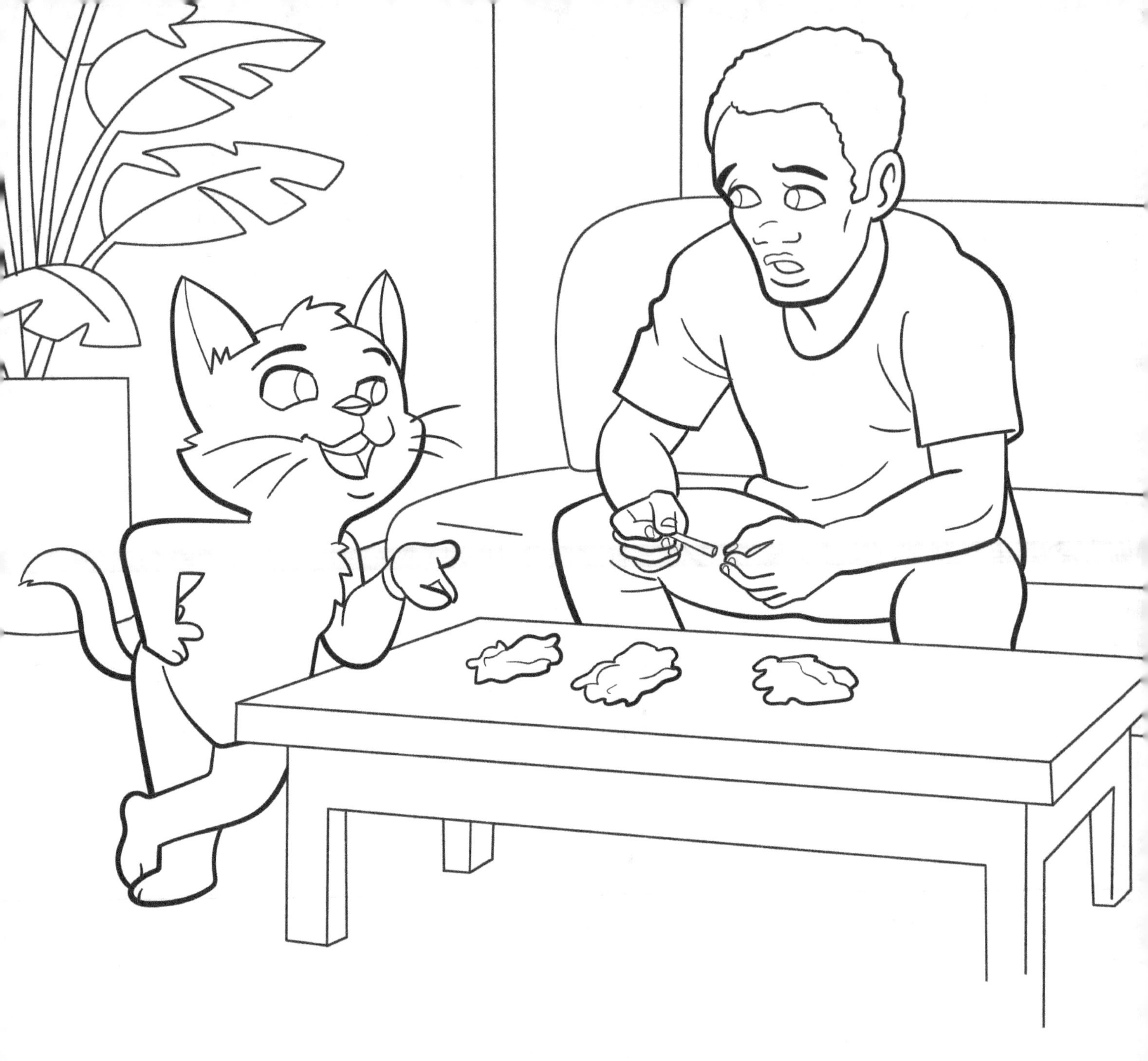

"These high THC strains will help you greatly. The Sativa will help you in the day and the Indica will help you in the evening before bedtime. The Hybrid is good for anytime," says Cannabis.

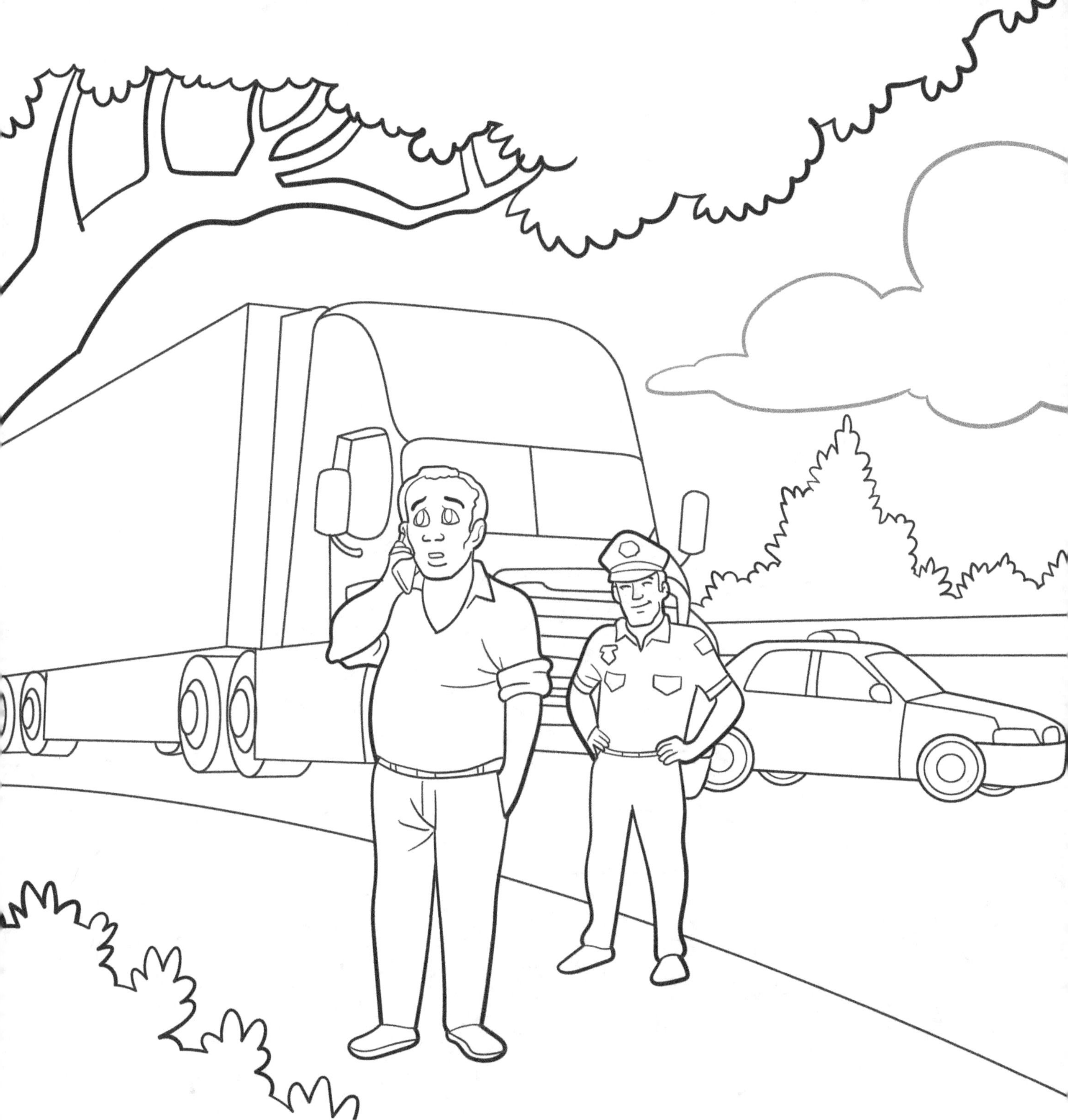

Seconds later, Cannabis's watch lights up. "This is Cannabis the Cat, what is your 420 emergency?"

"I'm a commercial truck driver, and my name is Phil. I'm hauling legal hemp (cannabis's cousin) across the state of Iowa, and I've been pulled over by the state police."

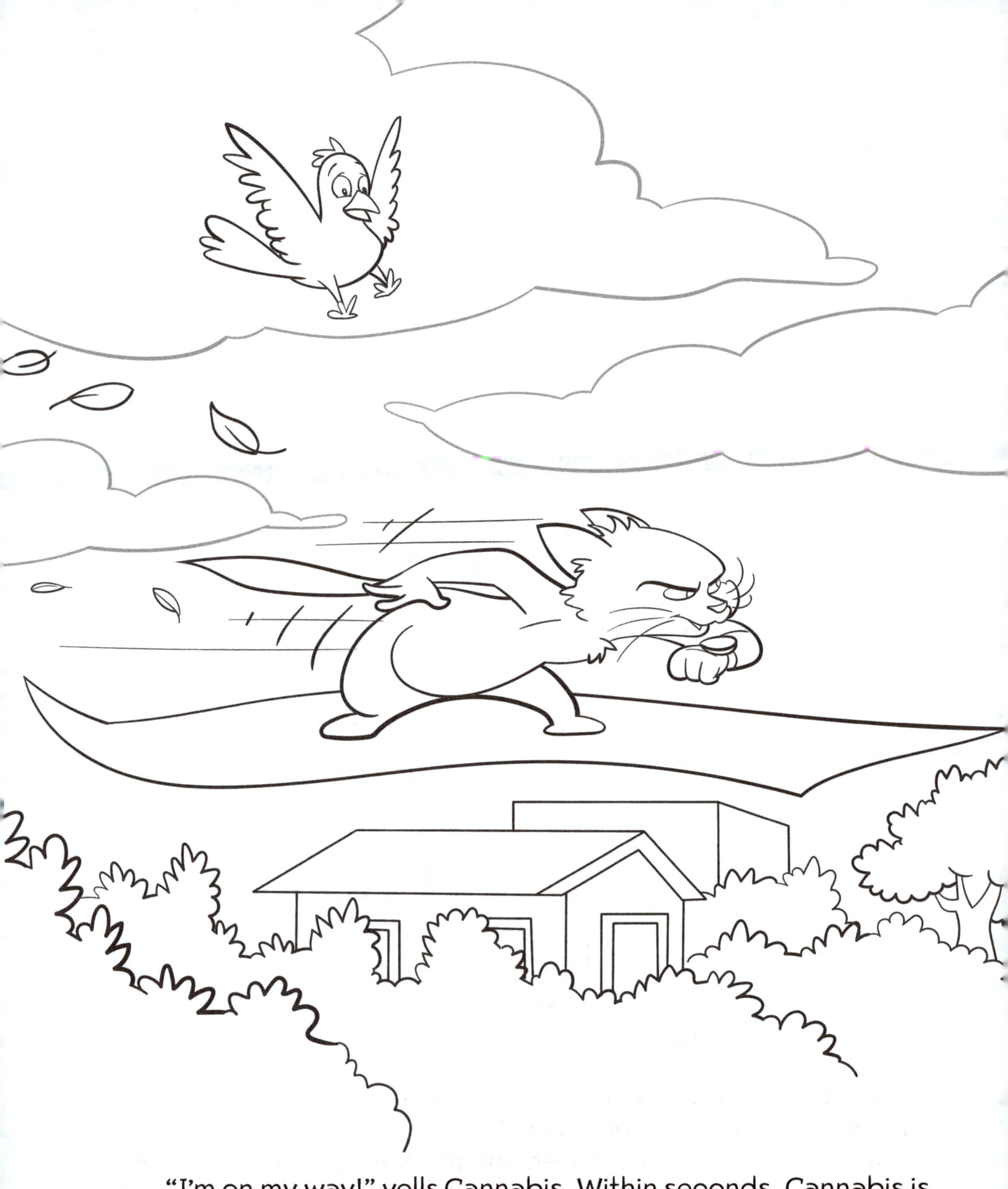

"I'm on my way!" yells Cannabis. Within seconds, Cannabis is flying in the air on his way to help Phil.

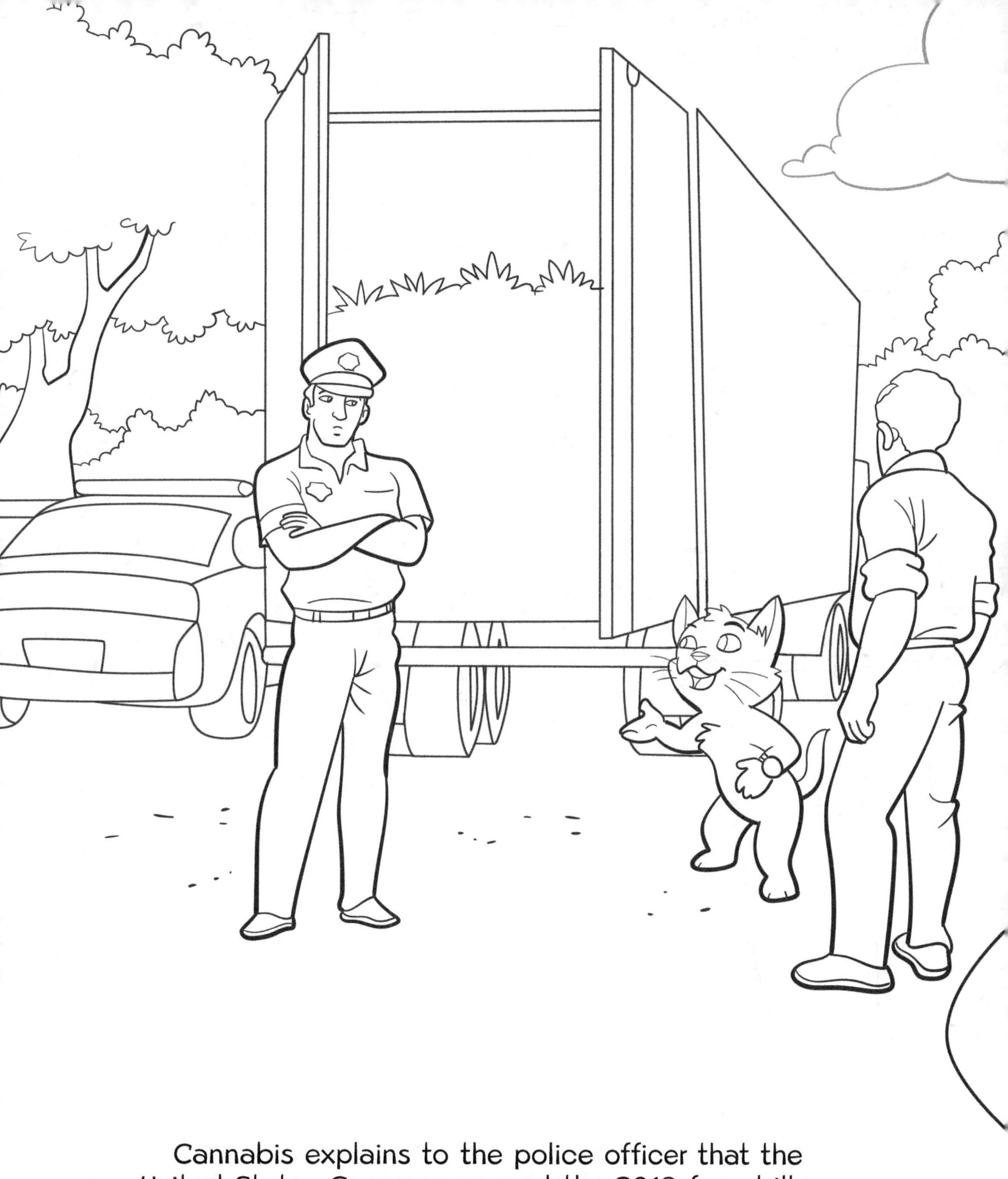

Cannabis explains to the police officer that the United States Congress passed the 2018 farm bill, and this legalized hemp in all 50 states.

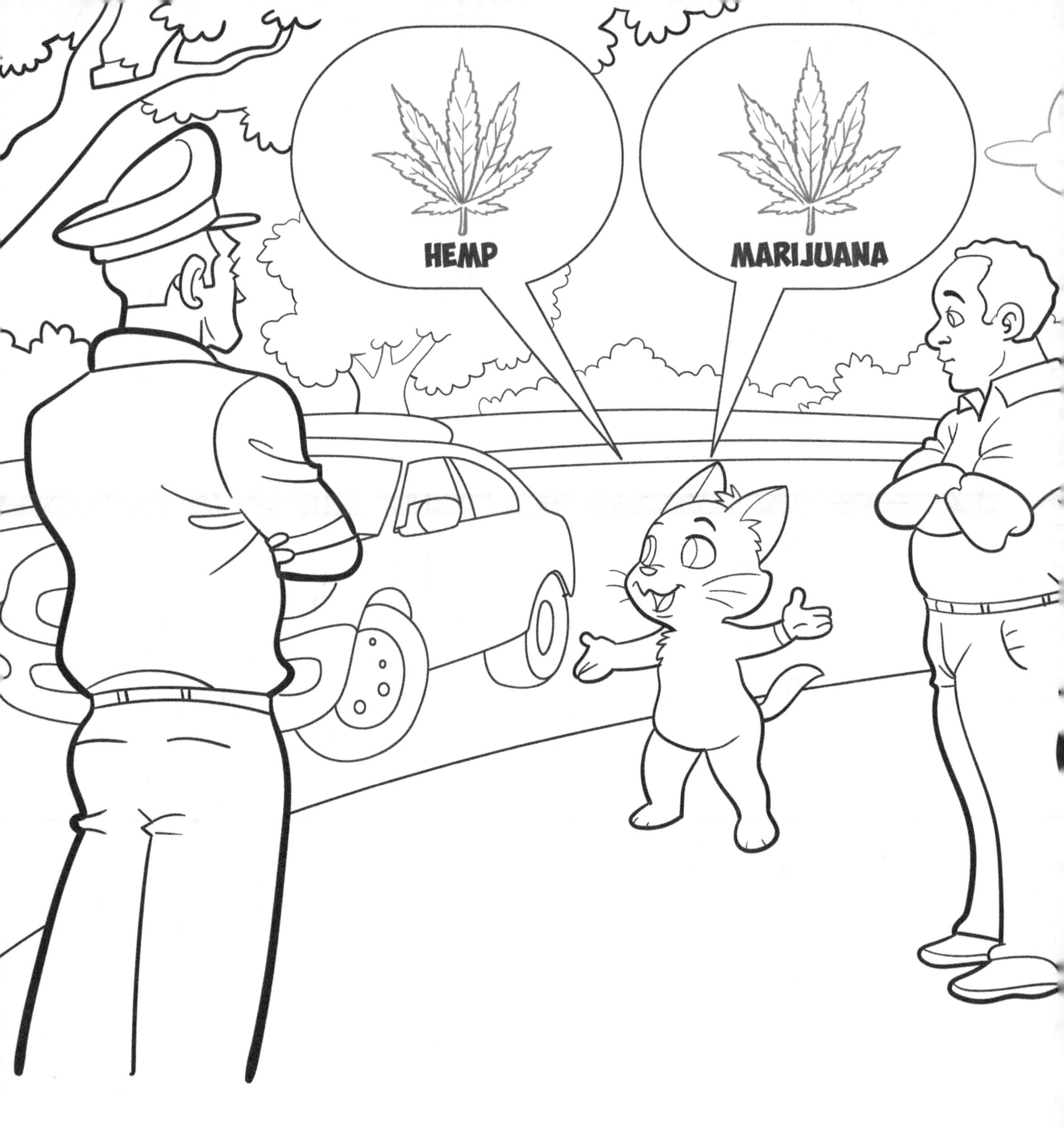

Cannabis points out that the hemp plant appears almost identical on the outside to the marijuana plant, but on the inside it's drastically different.

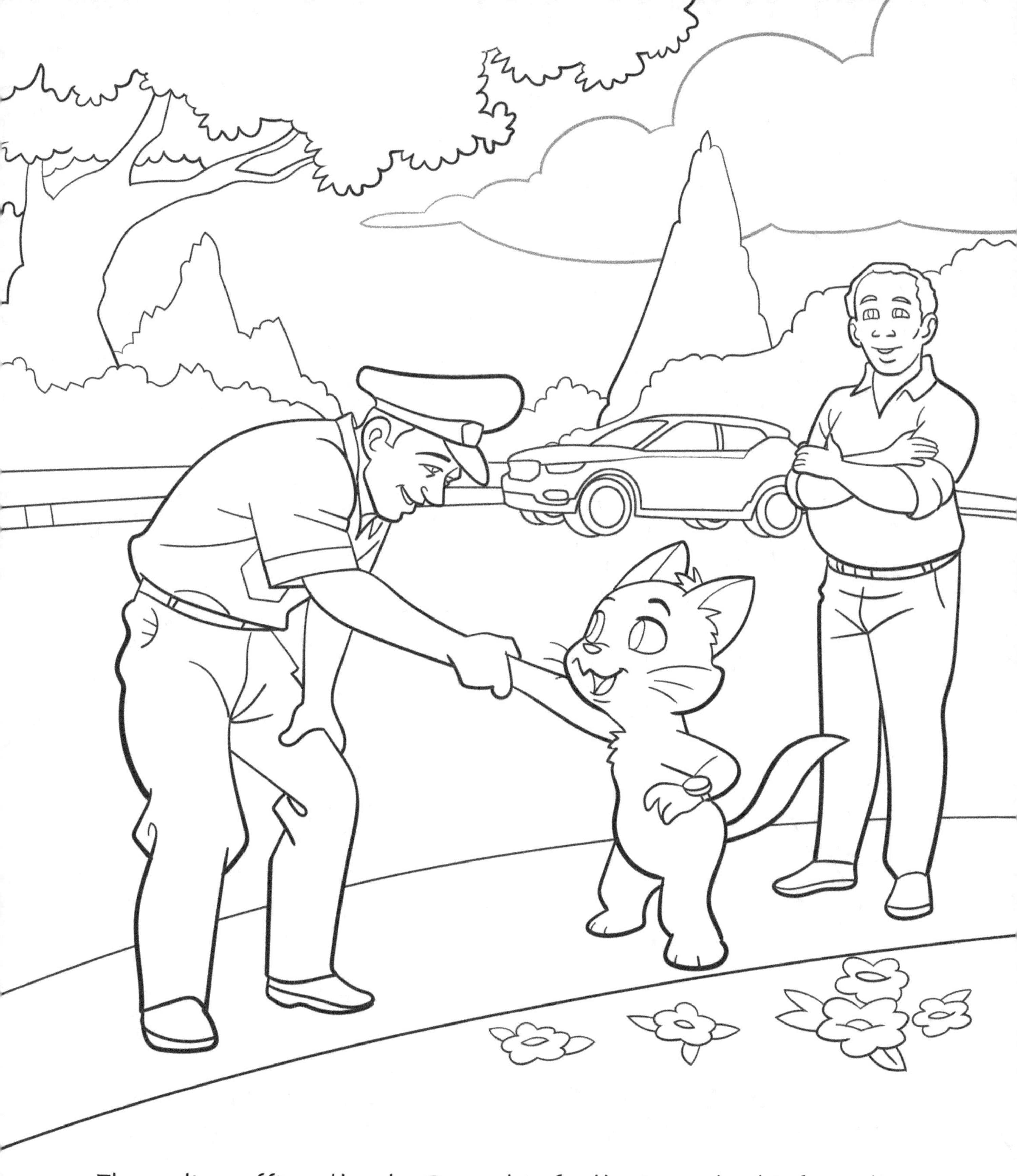

The police officer thanks Cannabis for the important information about the difference between hemp and marijuana.

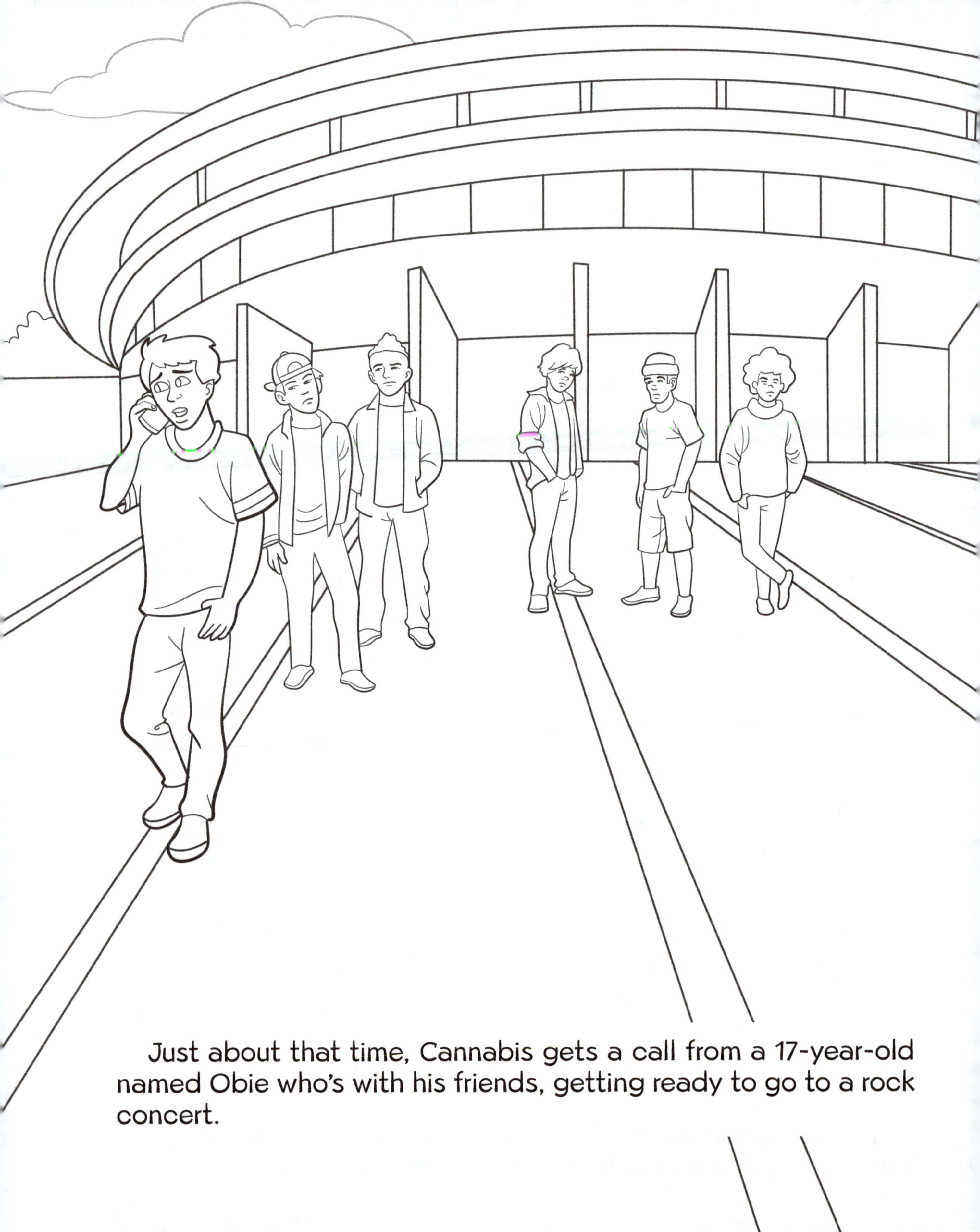

Just about that time, Cannabis gets a call from a 17-year-old named Obie who's with his friends, getting ready to go to a rock concert.

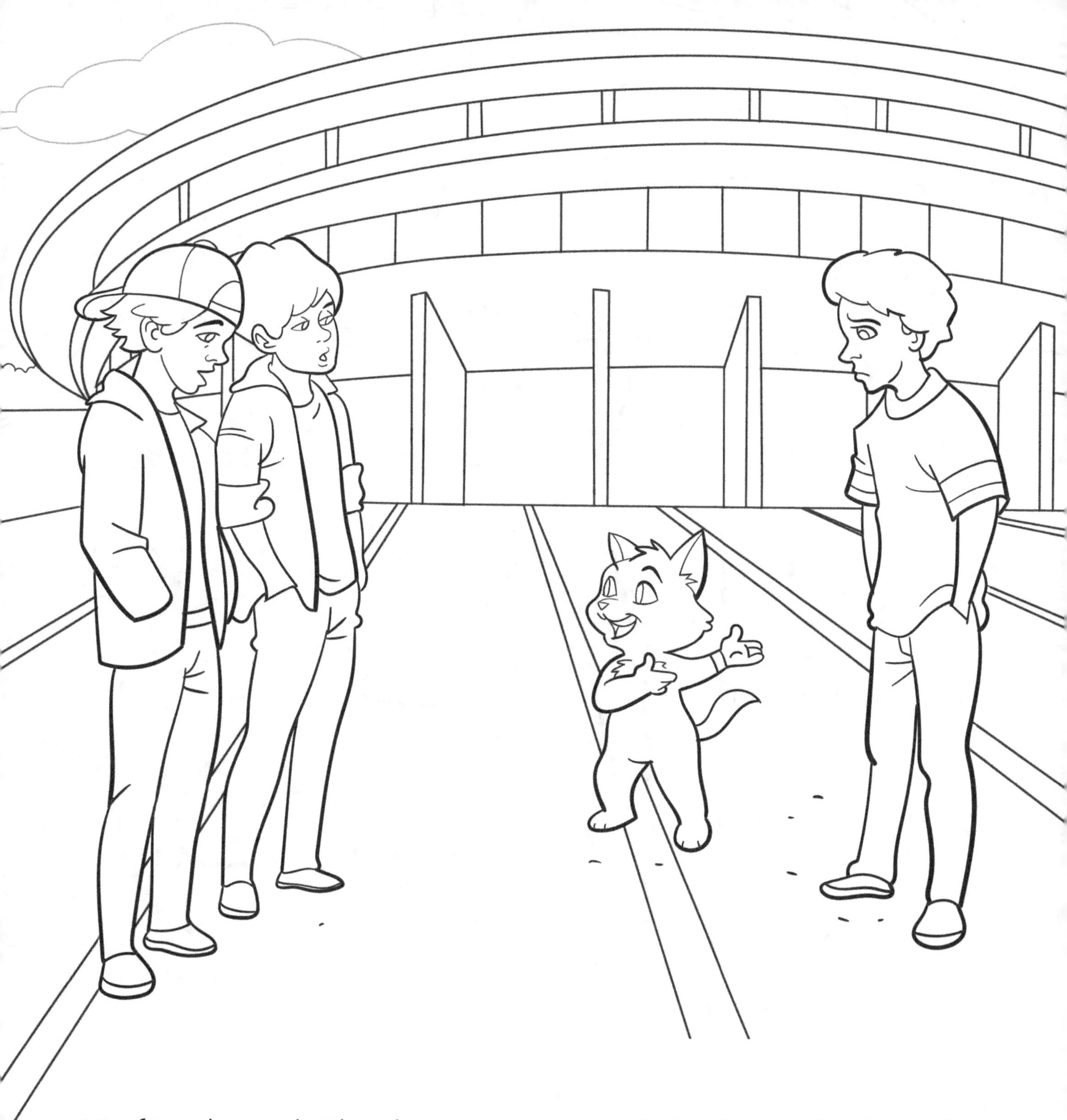

His friends want Obie to use marijuana, but Obie really doesn't want to. "Can you help them understand?" asks Obie. "I want them to still like me and be my friends, but I'm not interested in smoking weed."

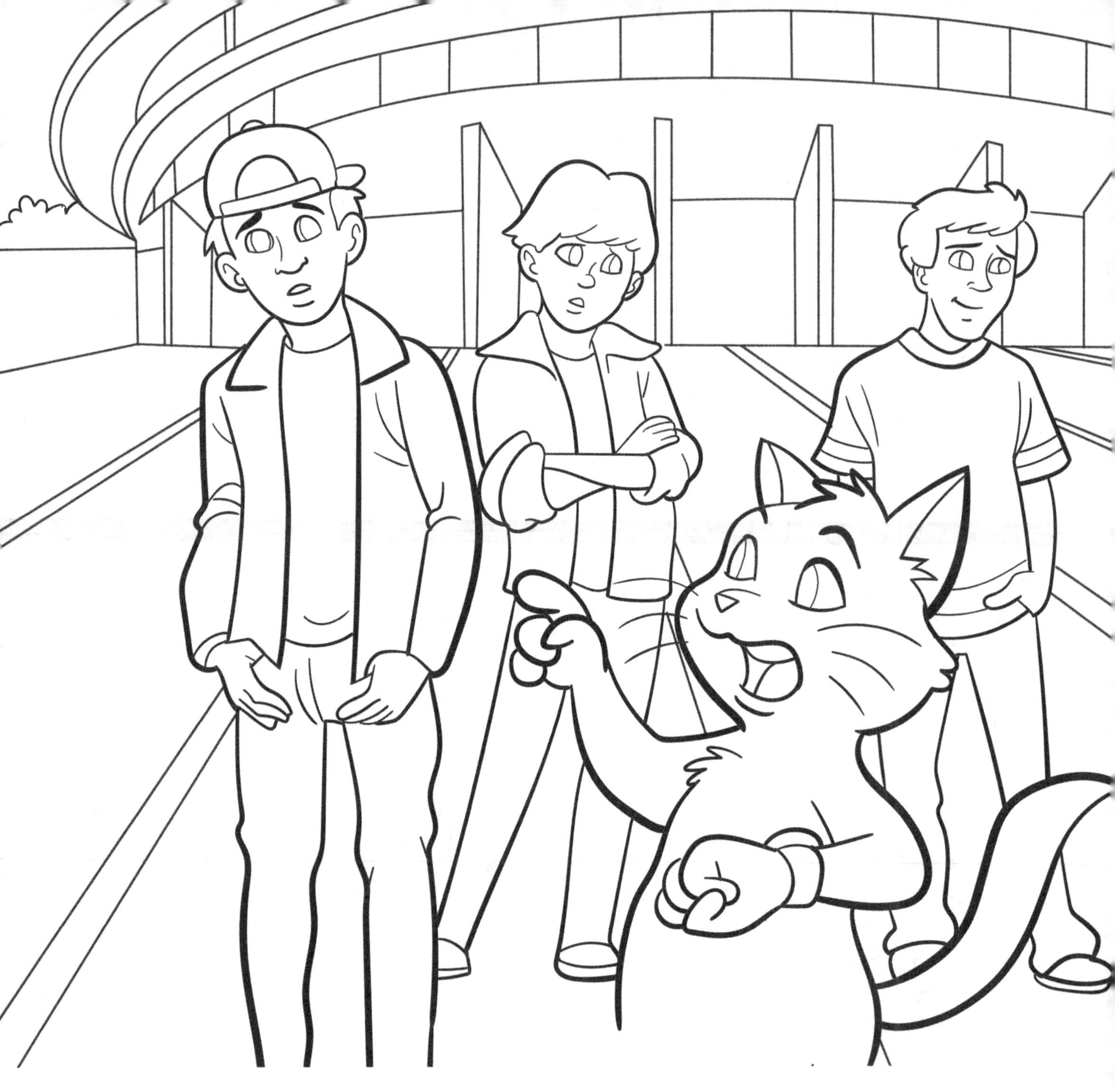

Cannabis explains to the boys the law says that you must be at least 21 years old for you to be able to consume marijuana legally. And never mix weed with driving an automobile. Cannabis leans in and reminds the boys that not everyone benefits from marijuana.

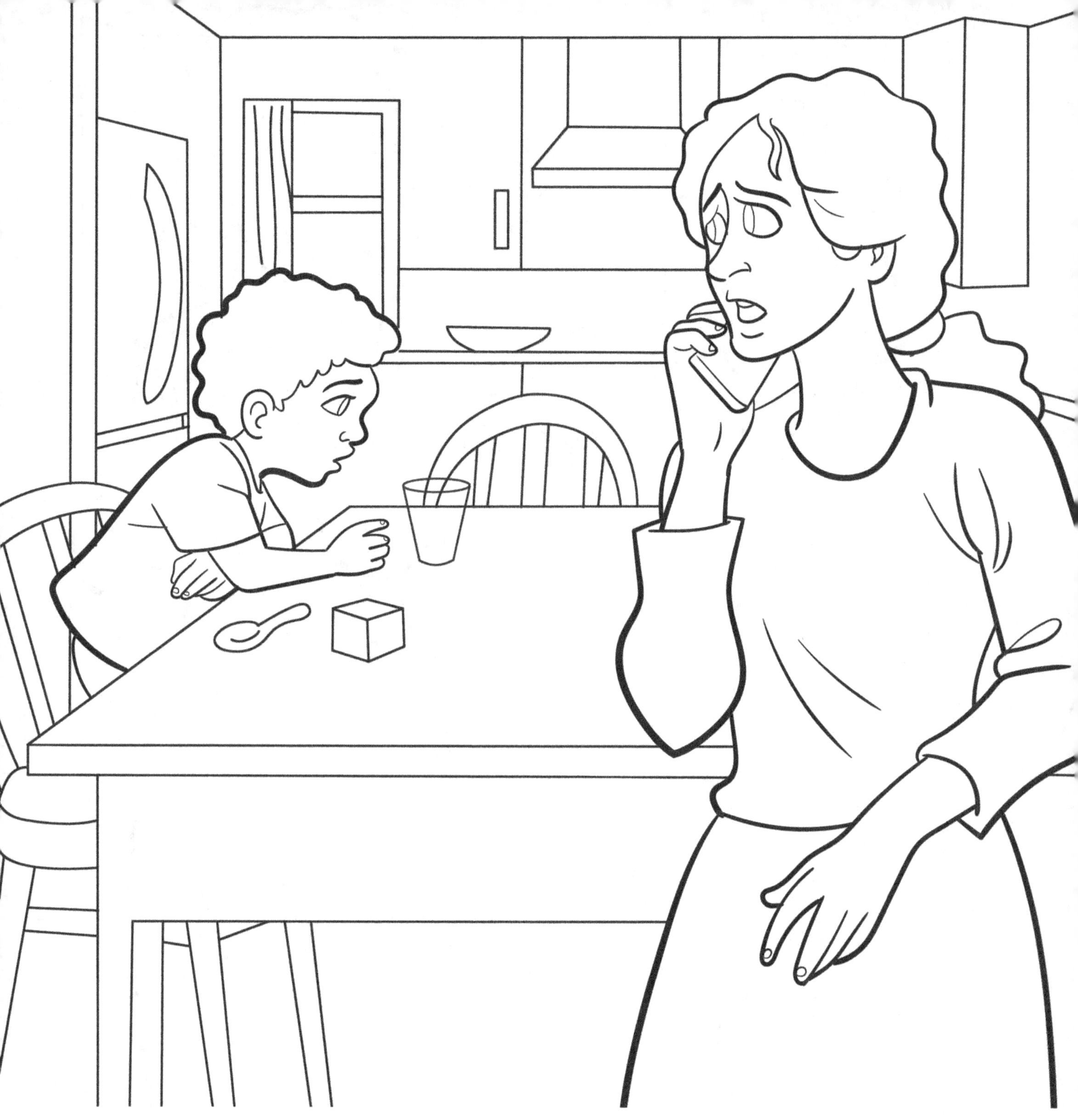

"This is Cannabis the Cat, what's your 420 emergency?"
"Hello, my name is Martina and my son, Carlos, is Autistic. I know for a fact that marijuana comforts him. Cannabis, can you tell us where we can legally buy marijuana edibles?"

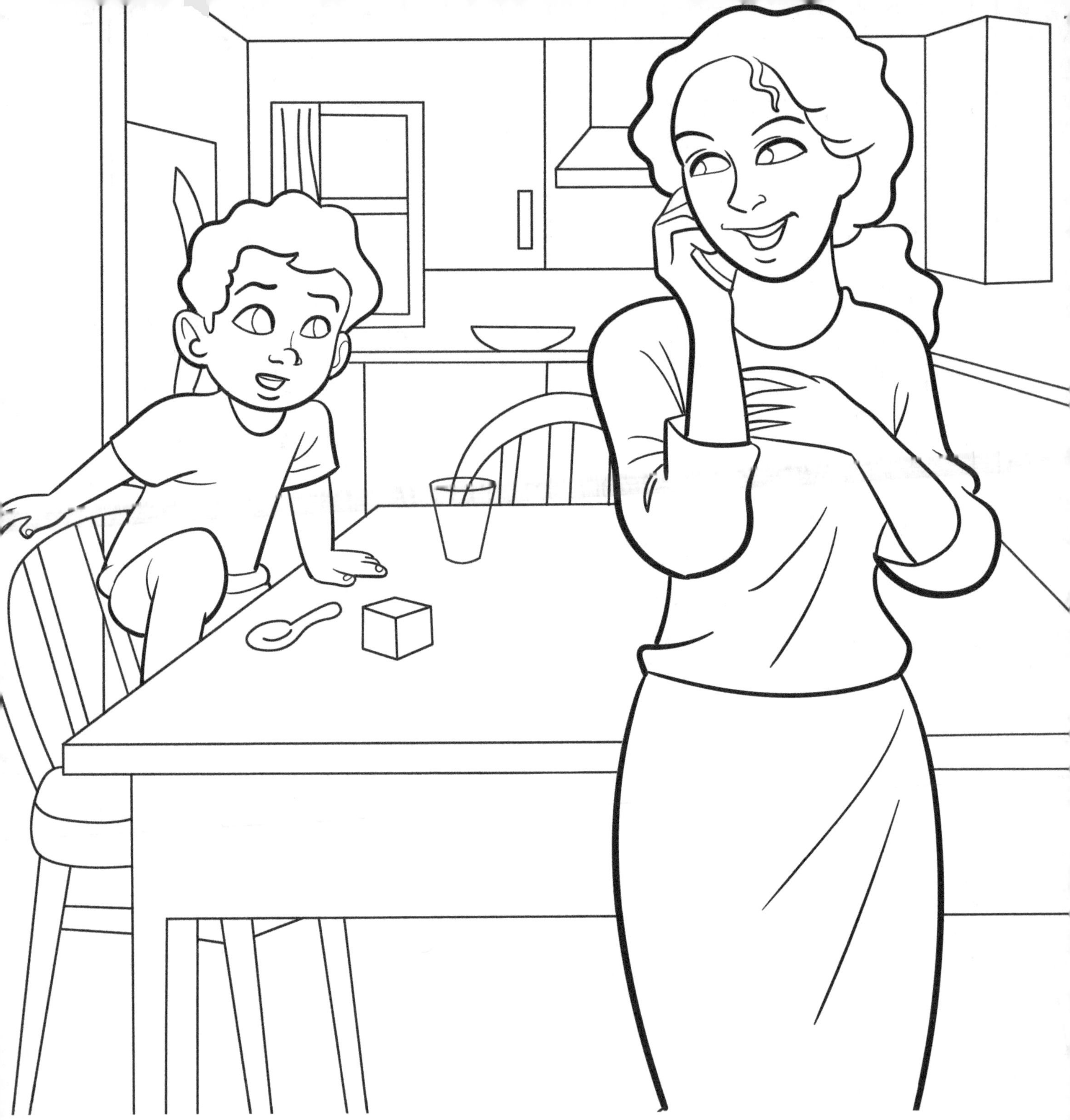

"Yes, of course. I will send you a list of legal marijuana dispensaries that are located close to your home."

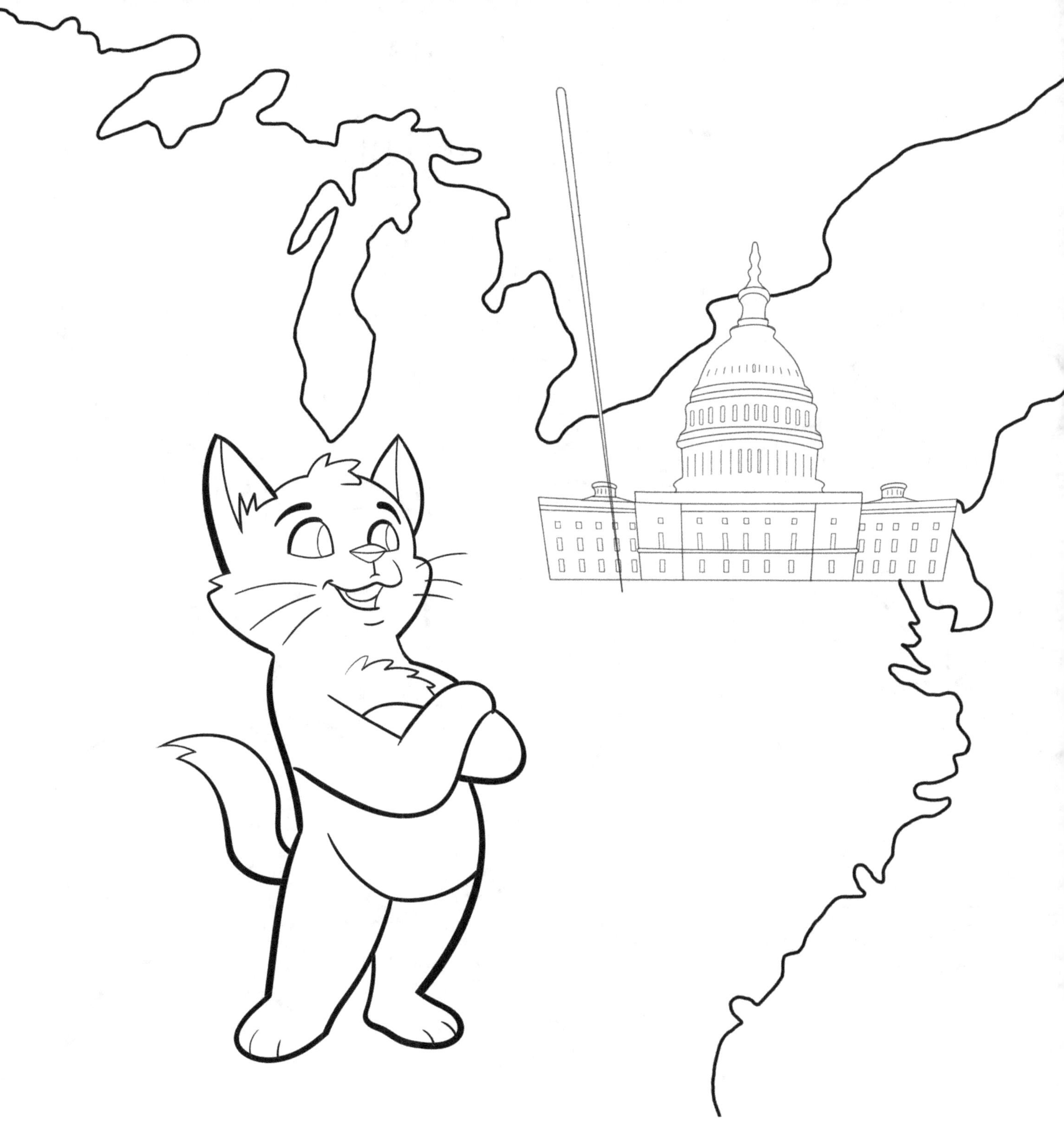

Cannabis gets ready for his big meeting in Washington, DC, this coming week. He will speak in front of US Senators and other important government officials about the usefulness of marijuana.

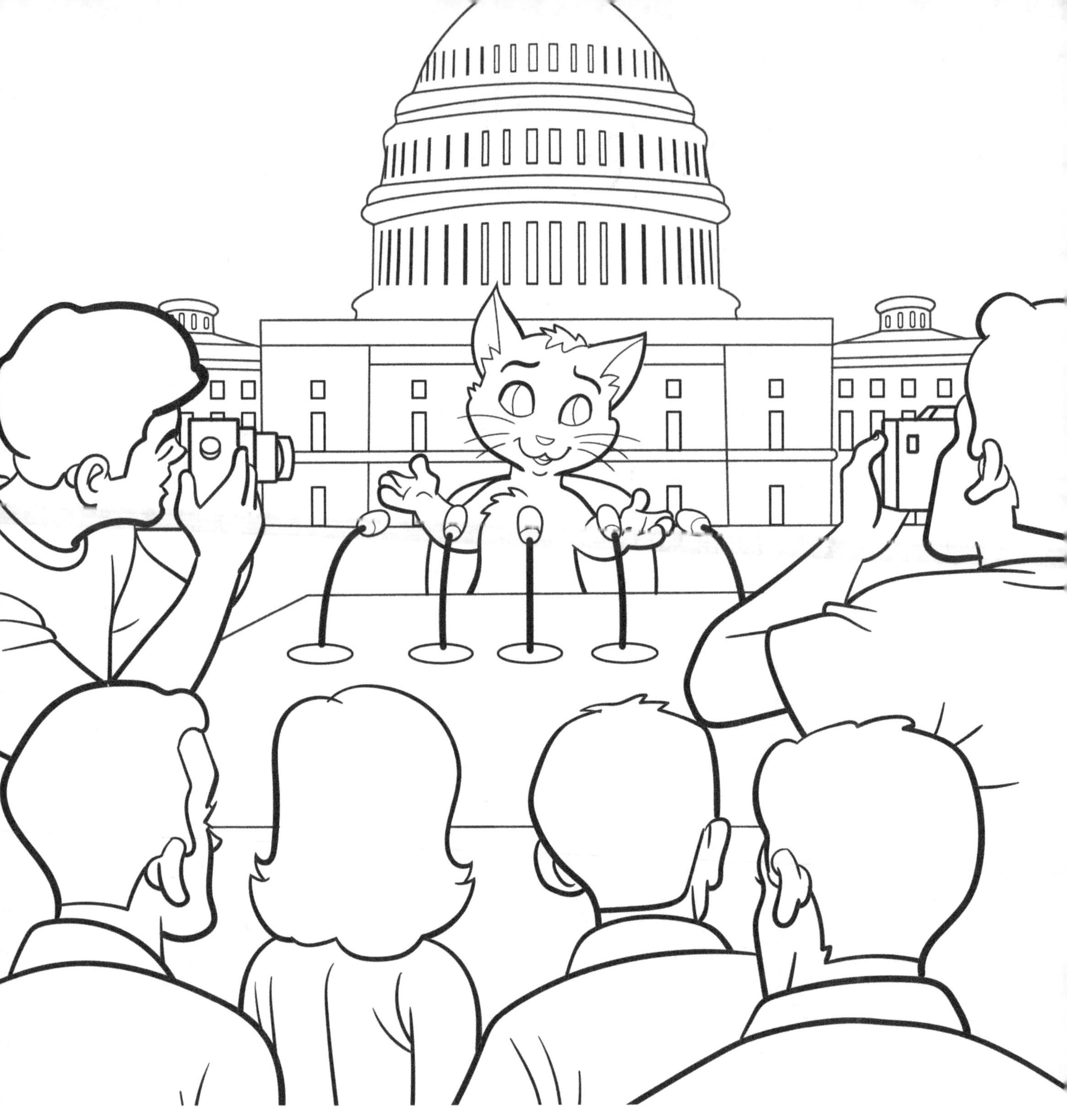

Once in DC, Cannabis quickly finds himself in front of cameras and microphones, where he tells stories about Charlotte, his friend in third grade who is seizure free because of CBD oil. And Devon, his veteran friend who gets great relief from his PTSD without using pills.

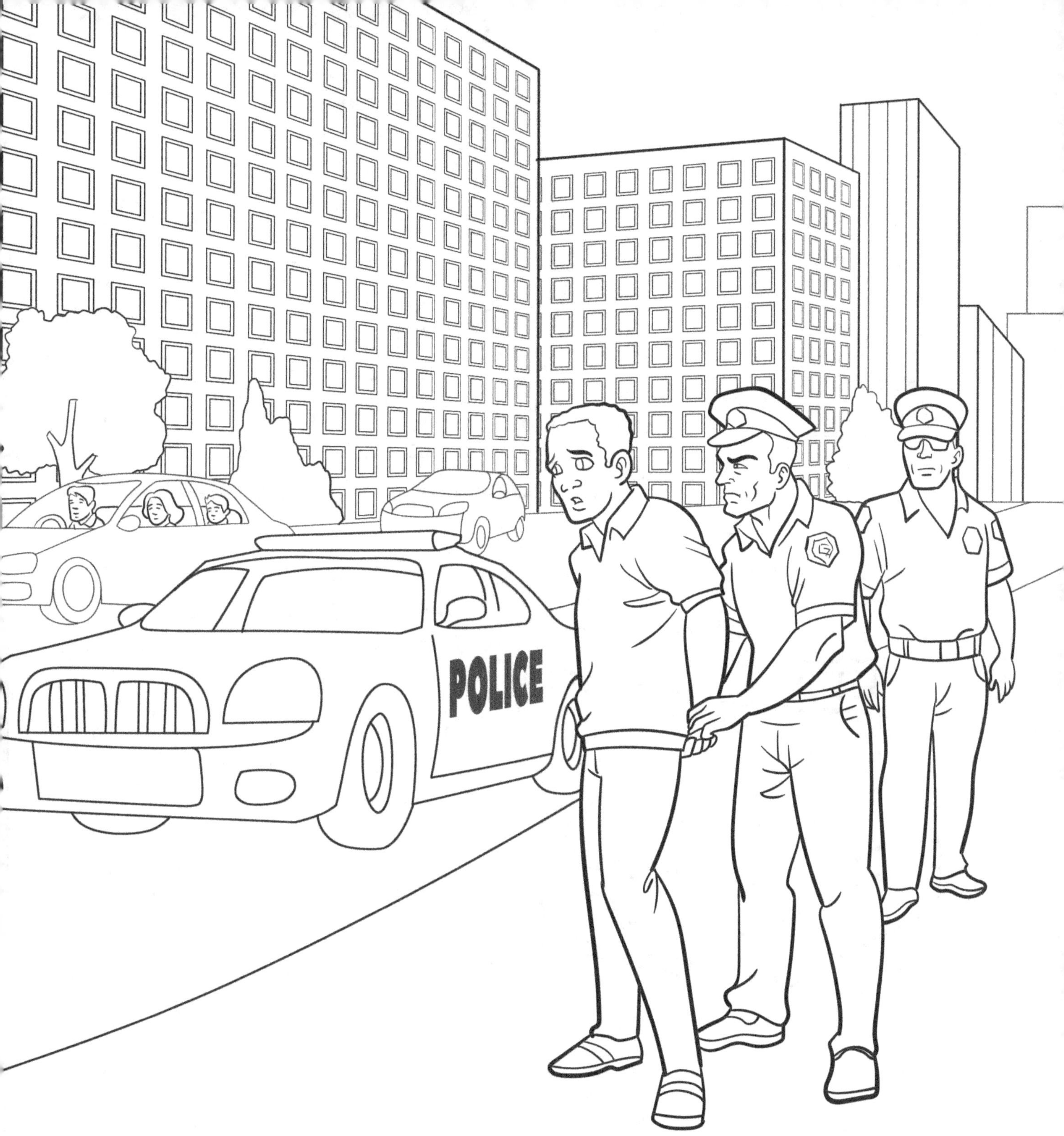

Cannabis lets people know about black Americans who are nearly four times as likely to be arrested for the possession of marijuana as compared to whites.

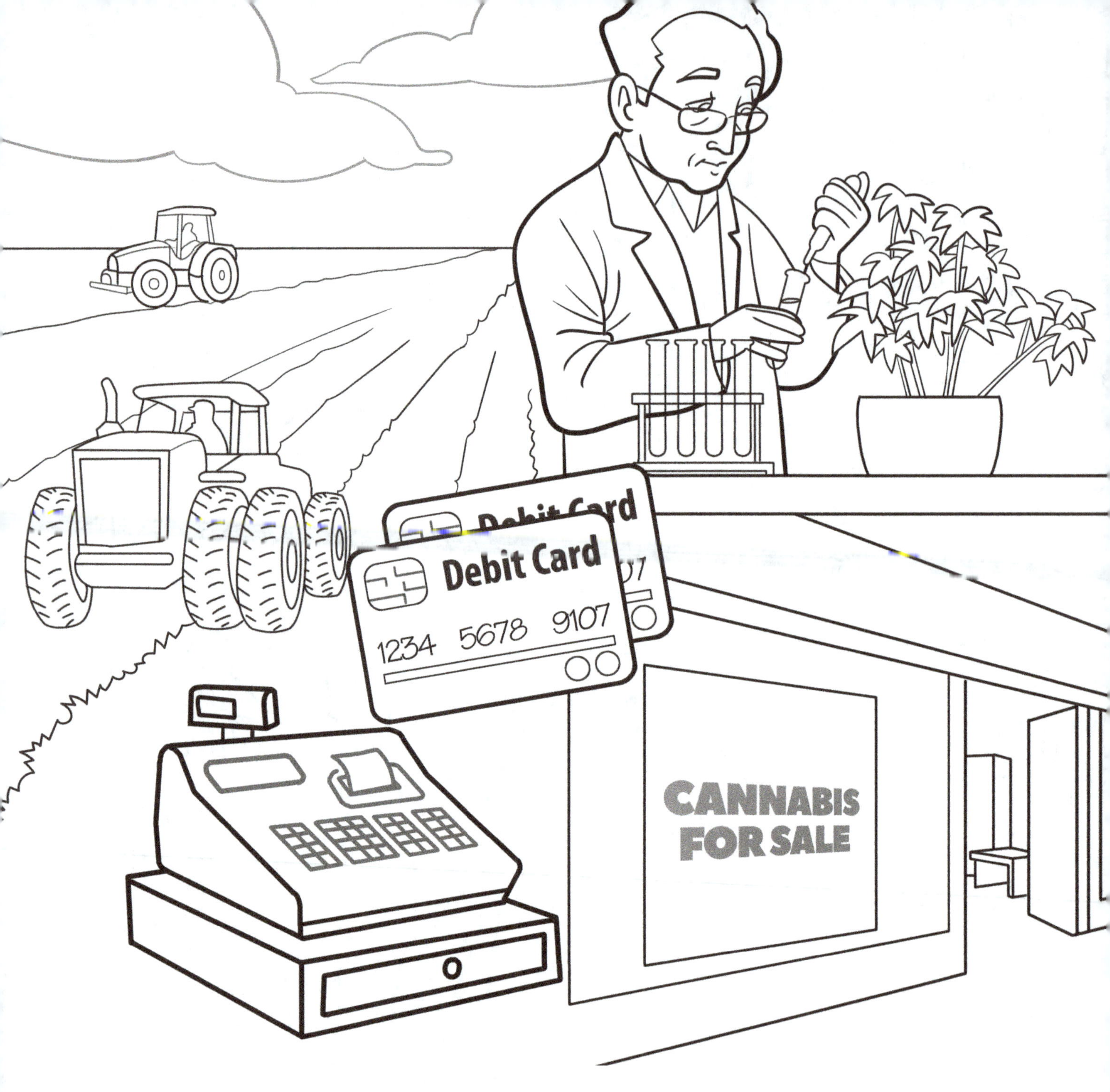

Cannabis stresses the need for us to deschedule marijuana and decriminalize it. This will create tens of thousands of new jobs and will also make it much easier for researching the plant.

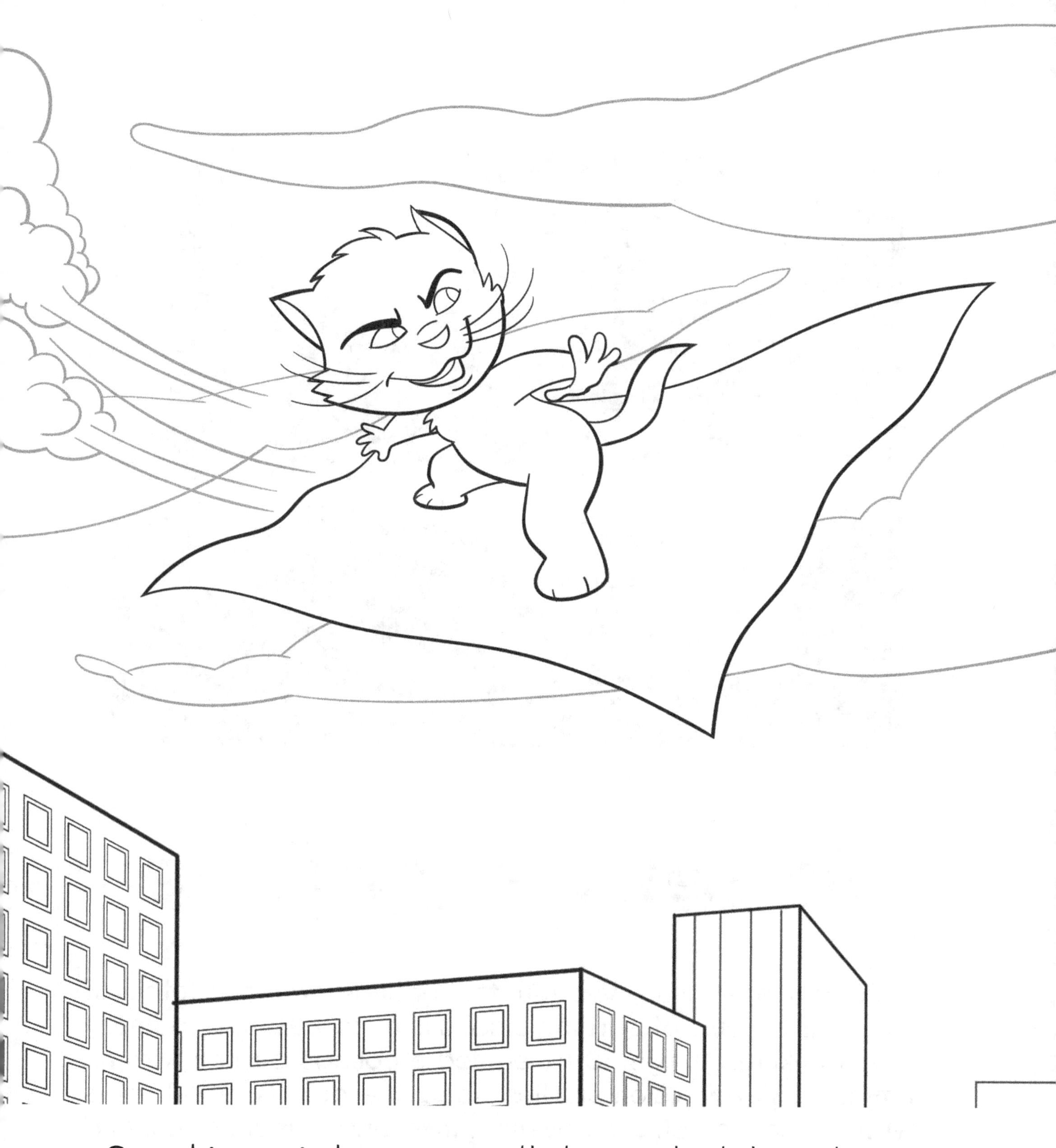

Cannabis reminds everyone that you don't have to use marijuana to love Cannabis the Cat. He then invites everyone to visit Cannabisthecat.com for his latest marijuana children's book *Cannabis the Cat to the Rescue!*

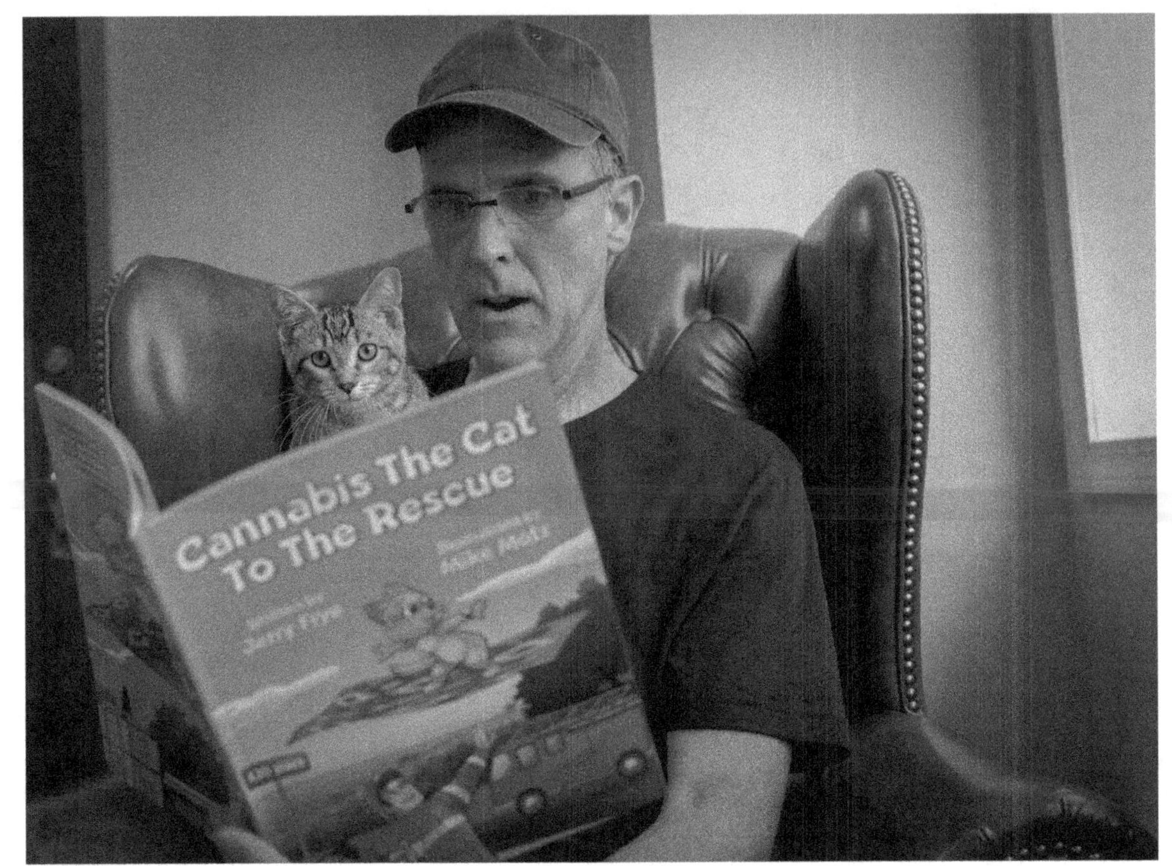

Meet Jerry Frye

Jerry Frye is a Navy veteran, former firefighter, and father of three. After years of battling alcoholism, he was able to finally stop drinking. At age 50 he earned a college degree with an emphasis in addiction studies. Today he celebrates 14 years without alcohol, enjoys traveling, investing in real estate, and lives with his cat named Cannabis.